Essential E

Essential Electromyography

John A. Jarratt
Emeritus of Sheffield Teaching Hospitals NHS Foundation Trust

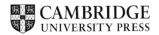
CAMBRIDGE
UNIVERSITY PRESS

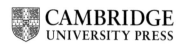

Shaftesbury Road, Cambridge CB2 8EA, United Kingdom

One Liberty Plaza, 20th Floor, New York, NY 10006, USA

477 Williamstown Road, Port Melbourne, VIC 3207, Australia

314–321, 3rd Floor, Plot 3, Splendor Forum, Jasola District Centre, New Delhi – 110025, India

103 Penang Road, #05–06/07, Visioncrest Commercial, Singapore 238467

Cambridge University Press is part of Cambridge University Press & Assessment,
a department of the University of Cambridge.

We share the University's mission to contribute to society through the pursuit of
education, learning and research at the highest international levels of excellence.

www.cambridge.org
Information on this title: www.cambridge.org/9781009381062

DOI: 10.1017/9781009381055

First published 2023

Printed in the United Kingdom by TJ Books Limited, Padstow Cornwall

A catalogue record for this publication is available from the British Library.

Library of Congress Cataloging-in-Publication Data
Names: Jarratt, John A., author.
Title: Essential electromyography / John A. Jarratt.
Description: Cambridge, United Kingdom ; New York, NY : Cambridge University Press, 2023. | Includes
bibliographical references and index.
Identifiers: LCCN 2023029575 | ISBN 9781009381062 (paperback) | ISBN 9781009381055 (ebook)
Subjects: MESH: Electromyography | Nerve Conduction Studies
Classification: LCC RC77.5 | NLM WE 560 | DDC 616.7/407547–dc23/eng/20230726
LC record available at https://lccn.loc.gov/2023029575

ISBN 978-1-009-38106-2 Paperback

....

To
Indy, Scarlett, Theo and Zachary
In the forlorn hope that they might be impressed.

Contents

Figures

Diagrams

Tables

Preface

The clinic where I first trained was called the Department of Applied Electrophysiology. No doubt the menace this implied of some junta-like operative extracting a diagnosis by whatever means necessary prompted a re-branding exercise. Departments of Clinical Neurophysiology sprang up, which seemed to place them within their natural neurological habitat and at the same time distinguishing them from the scientific hothouses of academic neurophysiology. There now seems to be a backward trend to label the specialty Electrodiagnosis or, consonant with the zeitgeist of social media, EDX.

This leads us to the difficulty in creating a title for this book. The name of the specialty would be an obvious choice but this cult of increasing concision is offset by its diminished allure. I hope that *Essential Electromyography* captures the aim of providing a brief account of the principles underlying the techniques involved in electromyography and nerve conduction studies rather than detailed descriptions of the techniques themselves. Changing fashions in nomenclature and even technique should not invalidate these principles.

An additional aim of the book is to introduce to a variety of readers what a professor of medicine once pejoratively if not condescendingly described to the author as the arcane world of clinical neurophysiology. This underlined what most practitioners of the specialty already know; namely, that many of their colleagues find the jargon as impenetrable as the basic principles underlying its exercise. With this in mind, an attempt has been made to describe or define technical terms when they are first encountered. A glossary is also provided.

The findings in commonly occurring conditions and how they are related to the underlying pathology are explained. The techniques involved are mentioned only where necessary and then briefly. In this way I hope the book will appeal not only to junior trainees in the subject but also to a wide range of clinicians such as neurologists, orthopaedic surgeons, general physicians, rheumatologists and endocrinologists who refer patients for investigation. This short summary should aid their selection of patients for referral and their appreciation of the implications of the results. Experience suggests that lawyers involved in medico-legal cases might also be interested.

Acknowledgements

It is a pleasure to thank my esteemed former colleagues Prof Tony Barker, Dr Arup Chattopadhyay and Dr Ros Kandler for all their support and wise counsel. I am grateful to the skilled artists in the Department of Medical Illustration at the Sheffield Teaching Hospitals for drawing many of the diagrams and for the kind permission from the Sheffield Teaching Hospitals NHS Foundation Trust to reproduce these images. I thank the team at Cambridge University Press, Anna Whiting, Camille Lee-Own, Beth Sexton, Reshma Xavier and Ursula Acton, who led this novice author through the daunting process of publication with understanding and professionalism.

Abbreviations

m/s	Metres per second.
ms Milliseconds	Also sometimes called msec. Thousandths of a second.
mV Millivolts	Thousandths of a volt.
μV Microvolts	Millionths of a volt.
ACh Acetylcholine	A chemical involved in transmitting impulses between nerves, and between a nerve and the muscle it supplies.
CMAP Compound muscle action potential	The potential recorded from a muscle after stimulating its nerve supply; representing the sum of all the individual muscle action potentials generated.
CNE Concentric needle electrode	A recording electrode produced by passing an insulated wire down the cannula of a hollow needle.
CV	Conduction velocity.
EPZ End-plate zone	The point at which a motor nerve connects to its muscle. See also NMJ, neuromuscular junction.
F-wave	A late and small compound muscle potential generated by antidromic stimulation of a motor nerve and subsequent firing of the anterior horn cell.
H-reflex	A late and small compound muscle action potential generated by orthodromic stimulation of muscle spindle afferents which connect monosynaptically to the anterior horn cell. Similar to a tendon reflex.
MAP Muscle action potential	The propagated potential generated by an active single muscle fibre.
MCV	Motor conduction velocity.
MNAP Mixed nerve action potential	The potential recorded from a mixed nerve representing the sum of the action potentials generated by individual active sensory and motor fibres.
MUAP Motor unit action potential	The potential generated by an active motor unit, representing the sum of all the individual muscle action potentials within that unit.
MUP	Same as MUAP.
M-wave	Same as CMAP.
NMJ Neuromuscular junction	The point at which a motor nerve connects to its muscle. See also EPZ, end-plate zone.
NMT Neuromuscular transmission time	The time taken for a nerve impulse arriving at the end-plate zone to generate a muscle action potential.
SAP Sensory action potential	Same as SNAP.
SCV	Sensory conduction velocity.
SNAP Sensory nerve action potential	The potential recorded from a sensory nerve representing the sum of the action potentials generated by individual active fibres.

Introduction

There are few difficult concepts in clinical medicine. Rocket science it definitely is not. But the bewildering profusion of nomenclature is undoubtedly a barrier to the understanding of many disciplines, clinical neurophysiology included.

Clinical neurophysiology is the application of electronic techniques to the nervous system and its connections for the purposes of diagnosis, monitoring and, occasionally, treatment. This book deals only with electromyography (EMG) and nerve conduction studies (NCS) as used in diagnosis and monitoring.

As with all diagnostic methods, be they purely clinical, or investigative or a combination, a number of general questions need to be addressed. These are listed here together with the issues specific to clinical neurophysiology:

- What is the location of the disorder? (Is it in muscle, nerve or the neuromuscular junction, and if in the nerve, is the condition local or widespread?)
- What is the pathology? (If muscle is affected, can it be defined? If nerve is implicated, is it degenerating, in which the nerve fibre itself is involved, or is it demyelinating, in which the insulating sheath around the nerve is damaged?)
- What is the severity and thus the prognosis? (What is the degree of change? And what is the likely clinical diagnosis and thus prognosis?)
- Having identified an abnormality, can it be monitored?

We start by defining the scope of the book. The first part deals with basic elements of anatomy, physiology and technical matters in an effort to provide some simple but sufficient background material. The second part then describes the principles of the examination methods and how they are used in clinical practice.

Peripheral nerves carry nerve impulses from the skin via the dorsal root ganglion to the spinal cord and thence to other parts of the central nervous system. These are sensory nerves. Nerve impulses to a muscle are sent from an anterior horn cell within the grey matter of the spinal cord to the neuromuscular junction from where they are transmitted to the muscle fibres. These are motor nerves. Both types are shown in Diagram 1.1.

Electromyography investigates disorders of neuromuscular transmission and also abnormalities within muscle arising from primary muscle disease or as a consequence of pathology within its nerve supply.

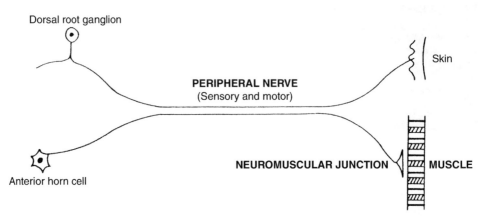

Diagram 1.1 An overview of the anatomical structures investigated by EMG and NCS. (Image included with permission from the Sheffield Teaching Hospitals NHS Foundation Trust.)

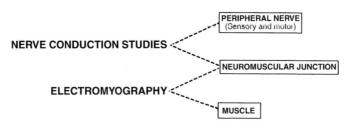

Diagram 1.2 An overview of the application of EMG and NCS to diagnosis. (Image included with permission from the Sheffield Teaching Hospitals NHS Foundation Trust.)

Nerve conduction studies are also used to investigate neuromuscular transmission. Their main function is to detect changes in peripheral nerves arising as a result of compression, or other forms of trauma, or systemic disease (Diagram 1.2).

The summary table, Table 1.1, outlines the plan of the text showing how these techniques are used in the clinic to try and answer the diagnostic questions posed earlier.

The completed table, Table 21.1, is given at the end of the book.

Table 1.1 A summary table outlines the plan of the book. The book concludes with its completion.

Anatomy	Pathology	Neurophysiology	
		EMG	*NCS*
Muscle	Myopathy		
Neuromuscular junction	MG		
	LEMS		
Peripheral nervous system		**D/M Neuropathy**	
	Compression lesions*		
	GPN***		
		D/G Neuropathy	
	Peripheral nerve lesions*		
	Plexus lesions**		
	Radiculopathy**		
	GPN***		
	AHC disease***		

Key to abbreviations:

* Local changes
** Regional changes
*** Widespread changes

MG Myasthenia gravis
LEMS Lambert–Eaton myasthenic syndrome
GPN Generalised peripheral neuropathy
AHC disease

D/M Demyelinating
D/G Degenerating

Basic Anatomy and a Little Physiology

The nervous system can be considered to consist of two parts: the central nervous system and the peripheral nervous system. A third component, the autonomic nervous system, features little if at all in the clinical application of electrophysiological testing. This and its complexity might permit us the notion that it should be enjoyed rather than understood.

The function of the individual elements, the neurons, of both parts of the nervous system is to transmit information from one site to another. Each neuron comprises a cell body, the soma, bearing an extrusion, the axon, which is usually of such impressive length that when referred to as a 'nerve' it is easy to overlook the fact that it is merely a conduit between the soma and its destination. Sensory neurons in the peripheral nervous system have two such axons and are therefore called bipolar cells.

The transmission of information may take place between sensory receptors and a neuron, between neurons or between a neuron and a muscle. The axon terminals from one neuron connect to the soma of another neuron at junctions called synapses. These are mainly located on dendrites, which are also extrusions of the soma but much shorter than the axon. A motor nerve connects to muscle fibres at the neuromuscular junction.

The brain and spinal cord comprise the central nervous system. Within this system, areas containing the cell bodies of nerves appear darker and are referred to as grey matter. At the base of the brain is a stalk-like structure, the brain stem, which forms a continuation of the spinal cord.

Grey matter in the brain is located over the surface, forming the cerebral cortex, or in clusters such as the thalamus and basal ganglia buried within the substance of the hemispheres. The grey matter in the spinal cord is deeply situated. It is roughly H-shaped having two ventral, or anterior, horns and two dorsal, or posterior, horns.

The interconnecting nerves between the cell bodies in the central nervous system are bundled into tracts known as white matter. They are sheathed in myelin which, containing lipids, imparts their lighter appearance. This insulates them from one another thus preventing unwanted 'cross-talk' between adjacent nerves. As we shall see in Chapter 4, 'Peripheral Nerve Function', the presence of myelin also increases the conduction velocity along the nerve.

Nerves supplying the limbs and trunk form the peripheral nervous system. The nerves to the head and neck have complex and individual anatomies and so rather than being thought of as a system, they are referred to by their individual cranial nerve names.

The majority of peripheral nerves are unmyelinated but in those that are, the myelin is applied in multiple, short segments.

Nerves carrying impulses into the central nervous system are called afferent or sensory nerves whilst those carrying impulses from the central nervous system to muscles are called efferent or motor nerves. Most but not all peripheral nerves contain some of both types of nerve and are therefore called mixed nerves.

Motor System

The motor nerves which supply the limbs and trunk arise in the cerebral cortex and then run through the part of the brain stem known as the medulla and thence down into the spinal cord where they form a synaptic link with the anterior horn cells in the ventral grey matter. Most of these fibres cross to the other side as they pass through the region of the medulla known as the pyramids to form the pyramidal or lateral corticospinal tract. The remainder form the anterior corticospinal tract.

The spinal cord, although a continuous structure, can be thought of as a sequential series of segments. The motor outflow from a given segment supplies a series of muscles, the myotome. The anterior horn cell pool of motor neurones supplying the myotome receives connections from the pyramidal tract and from the anterior corticospinal tract after it has decussated (crossed sides) at that level.

The nerves issuing from the anterior horn cells destined for the limbs and trunk exit from the spinal cord via the ventral nerve roots and then negotiate plexuses where sensory and motor nerves arising from different segmental levels in the spinal cord combine. Each paraspinal muscle receives its nerve supply from the dorsal ramus which arises just distal to the point where the dorsal and ventral roots at that segmental level merge.

The anterior horn cell, its peripheral nerve and all the muscles fibres it innervates is called a motor unit. The size of the motor unit is proportional to the number of muscle fibres it contains.

Sensory System

Sensory neurons within the peripheral nervous system are located in the dorsal root ganglia just outside the spinal cord. They differ from motor neurons in having not one but two extruded nerve fibres, hence the name bipolar cells. The peripheral, distal fibre brings in impulses from the limbs or trunk. It also participates with the motor nerves in the formation of plexuses. The centrally projecting fibre from the dorsal root ganglion runs into the spinal cord via the dorsal root and then follows one of two main pathways.

Nerves carrying pain, temperature and deep touch sensations cross the midline and form synapses in the posterior horns of the spinal grey matter. From here the lateral spinothalamic tracts relay signals to the cerebral cortex after making further synaptic connections in the thalamus.

Nerves carrying light touch and proprioceptive sensations do not cross the midline at this stage. They enter tracts called the dorsal columns which synapse in the cuneate and gracile nuclei located in the medulla. They then cross the midline in the medial lemniscus tract to the thalamus. Here they also engage in further synaptic activity before their onward journey to the cerebral cortex.

There is an exception to this general trend of relays mediated via multiple synapses. Nerves from the intrafusal muscle spindles, which signal information about its length, form a monosynaptic link with the anterior horn cells supplying the force-producing extrafusal fibres of the same muscle. This will be discussed further when we consider the H-reflex in Chapter 17, 'Other Techniques: F-waves and H-reflexes'. The intrafusal and extrafusal muscle fibres are discussed more fully in Chapter 6, 'Muscle'.

Soma, Axon Hillock and Initial Segment

We are now in a position to consider how an impulse from the spinal cord begins its journey to a muscle.

As we have seen, the soma – in this case, the anterior horn cell – has numerous small projections called dendrites and a long, extruded portion, the axon, which forms the peripheral motor nerve fibre. The activity in the connections between the axon terminals from other nerves and these anterior horn cell dendrites determines the activity of the soma and hence its nerve.

Neurotransmitters cross the junctions between these connection, the synapses, and induce either an excitatory or inhibitory potential in the soma. These are known as excitatory post-synaptic potentials (EPSPs) or inhibitory post-synaptic potentials (IPSPs), respectively. A single EPSP is insufficient to generate a so-called action potential in the axon, that is to say, a potential that will be propagated down the nerve. Both EPSPs and IPSPs may be augmented by spatial and/or temporal summation. In spatial summation, the effects of activity in multiple dendrites are summed. In temporal summation, the effects of repeated activity at a single dendrite are summed. The algebraic summations of the EPSPs and IPSPs then determine if the soma has been sufficiently depolarised to generate an action potential. If so, the soma is said to fire. How is this achieved? The currents from these potentials are routed to a bulge in the soma called the axon hillock from which the axon itself arises. The axon hillock and the so-called initial segment of the axon leading from it are both especially sensitive to depolarisation as they contain very high concentrations of sodium channels which facilitate the entry of sodium ions.

In this way, the soma weighs the evidence of incoming signals in determining whether or not to fire. When it does decide to do so, the physiology of the peripheral nerve means that there is no going back in either sense of the term. This relates to something called the absolute refractory period which, together with further details of the depolarisation process, will be described in Chapter 4, 'Peripheral Nerve Function'.

Peripheral Nerve Types

Peripheral Nerve Classification

Peripheral nerves were originally classified as A, B or C, in descending order of diameter. Nerve types A and B are myelinated; C is not. A more recent classification defines four subclasses of the A fibres, namely α, β, γ and δ, again in descending order of diameter. The Aα fibres are the efferents to the extrafusal muscle fibres; that is, fibres not within the muscle spindle. The Aγ fibres are the efferents to the muscle spindles. Afferent fibres within peripheral nerves now have a Roman numeral classification. The Ia fibres supply the annulospiral receptors of the muscle spindle; the Ib supply the Golgi tendon organ. Smaller diameter fibres, type II, supply the flower-spray endings in the muscle spindles and also the cutaneous mechanoreceptors. The smallest myelinated fibres within the group, type III, supply fast pain and cold receptors in the skin and also the free nerve endings subserving touch and pressure. Type IV fibres, the type C of the earlier classification, are unmyelinated fibres relaying sensations of pain and heat. These subtypes based on diameter/conduction velocity and function are helpful even though there is considerable overlap between the categories. Table 3.1 summarises the differences between them.

Nerves with the largest diameters, up to 20 microns (i.e. micrometres or μm), are found in the Ia, Ib and Aα categories. The smallest diameter fibres, of about 1 μm, belong to the unmyelinated type IV nerves.

Whilst it is important to have an appreciation of this classification, the message that needs to be kept in mind when performing nerve conduction studies is that peripheral nerves contain fibres of different diameters and these conduct at different speeds.

The detailed analysis of the behaviour of these different components of peripheral nerves falls within the remit of academic neurophysiology but a brief summary of the more pertinent aspects follows.

Sensory Nerves

Sensory nerves from the muscle spindles and tendons are designed to monitor muscle length and tension, respectively, and operate at the subconscious level. Sensory fibres supplying the muscle spindles, the Ia afferents, are the largest and fastest-conducting fibres in the peripheral nervous system. They provide information about muscle length and the rate of any change. They are relayed in the central nervous system to the cerebellum which co-ordinates movement. In the spinal cord, they also form a connection with the alpha motor neurons supplying the same muscle. If the muscle is stretched, they excite this alpha

Table 3.1 Peripheral nerve fibre types.

Fibre type	Myelination	Efferents	Afferents
Aα	Myelinated	Muscle extrafusal fibres	
Aγ	Myelinated	Muscle spindle	
	Unmyelinated		See IV
Ia	Myelinated		Muscle spindle annulospiral endings
Ib	Myelinated		Golgi tendon organs
II	Myelinated		Muscle spindle flower-spray endings and specialised receptors for touch, pressure and vibration
III	Myelinated		Mainly free nerve endings for fast pain and cold, and touch
IV	Unmyelinated		Mainly free nerve endings for slow pain, heat and cold

motor neuron to elicit a contraction thereby restoring muscle length. Because this reflex arc is based on one sensory neuron and one motor neuron it is called a monosynaptic reflex. And since this compensatory contraction would stretch antagonist muscles, the Ia afferents also form an inhibitory connection, via an interneuron, with the alpha motor neurons supplying them. The phenomenon is familiar as the tendon reflex of the knee-jerk. The tendons also contain receptors which signal muscle tension via the Ib afferents.

Other specialised cutaneous sensory receptors respond to specific stimuli such as pressure, vibration or light touch. Attempts to refine sensory nerve conduction studies by using modality-specific stimuli have not so far been clinically useful. Fortunately, there are abundant peripheral sensory nerves which can be easily stimulated to provide valuable diagnostic information.

Motor Nerves

The alpha motor neurons which arise in the ventral grey matter (also known as the anterior horn) of the spinal cord are responsible for muscle contraction. They are also fast-conducting nerves, only slightly less so than the Ia afferents.

More slowly conducting gamma motor neurons, which also arise in the ventral grey matter, supply the muscle spindles. They maintain tension on the spindle to match the desired length of the extrafusal muscle fibres. This is called alpha–gamma co-activation. Unintended departure from this state is signalled by the Ia afferents to the alpha motor neurons whose firing rates, which determine muscle tension, are correspondingly adjusted.

Peripheral Nerve Function

We now need to consider in more detail the structure of a peripheral nerve and how this relates to its functioning. The peripheral nerve has a semipermeable membrane. Outside the nerve, there is a predominance of sodium ions. Within the nerve, potassium ions predominate. An active energy-dependent process, the sodium–potassium pump, pushes out three potassium ions for every two sodium ions that enter. This leads to a resting membrane potential in which the interior of the nerve is approximately −70 millivolts (mV) relative to the exterior. Given that there is an excess concentration of sodium ions outside the nerve within a positively charged environment, one has to ask why the concentration and/or electrical gradients fail to propel them into the cell. One reason, but not the most important, is that sodium ions are hydrated, making them larger and so less diffusible. The other and critical factor is that entry of sodium ions takes place at specialised sites incorporating voltage-gated channels. These are ion channels which only open in response to specific changes in membrane potential. In the case of sodium ions, this is when the membrane is depolarised, that is to say, when the interior becomes more positive and the exterior becomes more negative.

If a peripheral nerve is stimulated as, for example, in a nerve conduction study, and if the stimulus strength is very low, the membrane will be depolarised but not sufficiently to produce a potential that will be propagated along the nerve. By definition, this is a subthreshold stimulus. But if the stimulus strength is sufficiently great to exceed the threshold, about 15 to 20 mV, the potential will be transmitted along the nerve. This is called an action potential and the nerve is said to fire. Once the threshold has been breached, many more local sodium channels are opened and the ions pour into the nerve, reducing the membrane potential even further.

As we have seen in Chapter 2, 'Basic Anatomy and a Little Physiology; Soma, Axon Hillock and Initial Segment', the depolarisation of the anterior horn cell and initial segment of the axon as a result of the opening of these sodium channels is well above threshold to produce an action potential.

Before we address the issue of how the action potential is then propagated along the nerve, we need to reflect a moment on peripheral nerve structure. Some, but not most, of the peripheral nerves are myelinated and since these are the ones we study in the clinic, they are the ones we consider first.

Diagram 4.1 shows a myelinated nerve fibre at low-power magnification and, below it, cross-sectional and longitudinal sectional diagrams at higher magnification. In reality, myelin appears as concentric rings in a cross-sectional view, which the author hopes will justify the artistic licence in depicting it as such.

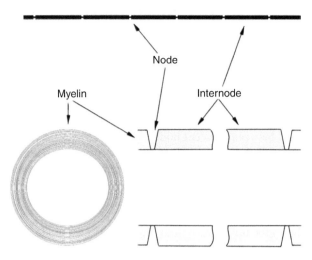

Diagram 4.1 Low-power and high-power representations of a myelinated nerve fibre. (Illustration by author.)

Schwann cells containing myelin and lying adjacent to the axon wrap around it rather in the manner of a Swiss roll. Between each cell, the axon is exposed at the node of Ranvier. If an additional foodstuff metaphor is allowed, a myelinated nerve resembles a string of sausages. The density of the voltage-gated sodium channels is especially high at the nodes.

The myelin segments between each node greatly facilitate the flow of sodium ions along the interior of the nerve rather than across its membrane. Two factors account for this. First, the myelin increases the resistance of the nerve membrane, thus reducing the outward flow of sodium ions. Second, the structure and fatty composition of the myelin sheath reduce the electrical capacitance of the membrane. If we have two conducting media, in this case the internal axoplasm within the nerve and the external extracellular fluid, which are separated by an insulating material, the myelin, then from $q = CV$ where q = charge (i.e. current × time), the voltage (V) across the nerve membrane is determined by the charge on it divided by its capacitance (C):

$$\text{voltage} = \frac{\text{current} \times \text{time}}{\text{capacitance}} \quad \text{or} \quad \text{time} = \frac{\text{capacitance} \times \text{voltage}}{\text{current}}.$$

If the capacitance is reduced, then the time to reach the depolarising voltage from a given current will be reduced. This means that the conduction velocity will be increased. We can now review what happens at the depolarised node.

The massive and self-perpetuating increase in sodium conductance is short-lived. As it is switched off, a slower but more sustained outward potassium conductance takes over. This not only restores the membrane potential but, because of its relatively long duration, there is a brief overshoot period during which the membrane becomes slightly hyperpolarised.

The inward rush of sodium ions lasts only one or two milliseconds. It is halted by the sodium channels becoming inactivated. During this period of inactivation no stimulus, however strong, will depolarise the nerve. This is called the absolute refractory period and normally lasts three to four milliseconds. After that, two opposing factors come into force. On the one hand, sodium channels progressively regain their activity, favouring a return to normal excitability. On the other, potassium conductance increases, driving the membrane potential towards normal and, as described, for a short time hyperpolarising it. Between the end of the absolute refractory period and the recovery of the normal resting potential, the nerve can be activated again but the stimulus required to do so is greater than that normally required to exceed the threshold potential. This period is called the relative refractory period.

While this is happening, the positively charged sodium ions that have entered the nerve are moving along its interior in both directions to the next nodes. This causes depolarising currents to be created between adjacent nodes. However, the refractoriness of the recently depolarised node means that the only node that can now be depolarised is the next one along in the direction of the propagated potential. The refractory periods therefore act as a kind of valve, ensuring that physiologically generated action potentials travel only in the intended direction. It is also clear that the duration of the absolute refractory period governs the maximum firing frequency of the nerve.

Diagram 4.2 shows the influx of sodium ions at the active node, **A**. Sodium ions then travel in both directions along the axon. This causes a reduction in the membrane potential. However, at node **B**, the sodium gates have been closed and the nerve at this point is in its absolute refractory state. At node **C**, however, the depolarising effect of the positively charged sodium ions is sufficient to open the sodium channels to allow more sodium ions to cascade into the nerve and thus continue the propagation of the action potential.

The presence of myelin segments around the peripheral nerve causes the depolarising current to jump from node to node. This is called saltatory conduction, from the Latin – dance, leap or jump. This has two benefits. It increases conduction velocity and, since the conduction process itself is energy dependent, it is more efficient. It should be added here that conduction velocity is also proportional to nerve fibre diameter. This is because a wider fibre presents less resistance to the internal flow of sodium ions.

Unmyelinated fibres have abundant sodium channels throughout their length. But as the depolarisation process proceeds from one channel to the next, it is clear that conduction velocity is very much slower than in myelinated fibres. This type of conduction is known as continuous conduction.

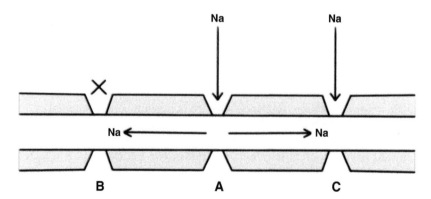

Diagram 4.2 The flow of sodium ions along a myelinated nerve during impulse transmission. (Illustration by author.)

In peripheral motor nerves, the impulses travel from the spinal cord to the muscle. In sensory nerves, impulses travel from the periphery to the central nervous system. These physiological directions of travel are called orthodromic conduction.

When we stimulate a peripheral nerve, the wave of depolarisation spreads in both directions. In the case of a motor nerve, impulses which travel towards the muscle, as they would physiologically, are conducting orthodromically; those travelling in the opposite direction towards the spinal cord are said to be conducting antidromically. Similar considerations apply, of course, to sensory nerves.

Chapter 5

The Neuromuscular Junction

A motor nerve divides into fine nerve terminals, each one innervating a single muscle fibre at approximately the mid-point along its length. The narrow region of the muscle encompassing these terminals is called the end-plate zone.

The terminals, which are unmyelinated, exhibit a swelling at the tip called the synaptic bulb. This fits into a corresponding cavity in the end-plate region of the muscle, which is thrown into many so-called junctional folds to increase its surface area. The gap between the synaptic bulb and the muscle is called the synaptic cleft, as shown in Diagram 5.1.

Within the synaptic bulb are large numbers of membrane-bound, spherical structures called vesicles which are packed with acetylcholine (ACh). Under resting conditions, a few vesicles become attached to the synaptic bulb membrane which then opens up to allow the contents of the vesicles to be discharged into the synaptic cleft. The process is known as exocytosis. Acetylcholine in the cleft quickly attaches to the nicotinic acetylcholine receptors lining the junctional folds. The receptors are sodium channels which open when bound to ACh. Entry of sodium ions causes depolarisation of the muscle membrane. But these small, spontaneously occurring potentials, which are called miniature end-plate potentials, are insufficient in size to generate an action potential. However, when a nerve action potential invades the nerve terminal, it triggers an avalanche of calcium ions to enter the synaptic

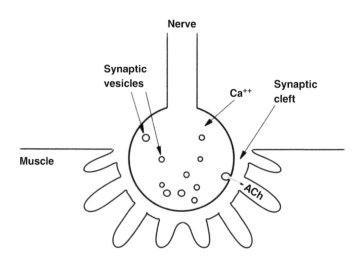

Diagram 5.1 Basic structure and function of the neuromuscular junction. (Illustration by author.)

bulb. The massive consequent release of ACh binds to the muscle receptors causing entry of sodium ions in sufficient numbers to generate a muscle action potential; that is to say, a potential which is propagated along the muscle fibre. The placement of the end-plate at the mid-point along the length of the muscle ensures that all parts of it are depolarised in the shortest possible time. The amount of ACh released is normally much more than required, a concept known as the safety factor. Afterwards, ACh is broken down by acetylcholinesterase into its constituent components, of which choline is re-absorbed into the nerve terminal for re-use.

The faster the firing rate of the motor axon, the greater and more sustained the muscle force. Which is interesting because, as we have seen in Chapter 2, 'Basic Anatomy and a Little Physiology', the anterior horn cell fires only when the combined inputs at its dendrites are strong enough to depolarise it. This could be regarded as an analogue to digital conversion. At the neuromuscular junction, the relationship between motor nerve firing rate and the force of muscle contraction could then be thought of as a digital to analogue conversion. Perhaps.

Muscle

Limb muscles consist of extrafusal and intrafusal fibres. The former are larger in diameter and generate the motive force of the muscle. The intrafusal fibres, also known as the muscle spindles, are smaller in diameter and fewer in number. By providing information about the degree and rate of change in muscle length, they assist in maintaining desired muscle tension.

Extrafusal Muscle Fibre Types

Within muscles of the human body, three types have been identified. The criteria for their differentiation are principally concerned with their twitch speeds, and also their metabolism and thus their fatiguability.

At one extreme, we have the slow oxidative fibres, type 1. These oxidise glucose to produce the high energy ATP (adenosine triphosphate) required for muscle contraction. To enable this, they are rich in mitochondria and also myoglobin, which binds the oxygen locally. The muscle fibres, which are of small diameter, contract relatively slowly and produce modest force but are resistant to fatigue.

At the other extreme, there are the fast glycolytic fibres, type 2b. They are large diameter fibres that can produce ATP rapidly by anaerobic (i.e. non-oxidative) glycolysis. These muscles have fast twitch tensions and can produce great force but fatigue relatively rapidly. They contain small numbers of mitochondria and amounts of myoglobin.

The remaining intermediate fibres, type 2a, are the fast oxidative fibres. Their fibre size, twitch tensions, force production and fatiguability are intermediate between the other two. Their metabolism is largely but not entirely oxidative. Table 6.1 summarises these differences. Human muscles contain all three types but principally types 1 and 2b.

All muscle fibres within a motor unit are of the same type. This is also true of the muscle fibres adopted by a regenerating motor unit during collateral re-innervation which, if necessary, change their type. The process of collateral re-innervation is discussed in Chapter 10, 'Electromyography; Motor Unit Size'. Histologically, the changes appear as fibre-type grouping. It should be appreciated that the cross-sectional area within a muscle occupied by the muscle fibres of one motor unit are intermingled with those from many other motor units.

Muscle Contraction

Depolarisation of the end-plate results in a massive influx of calcium ions into the muscle tissue. This in turn causes the two filaments within the extrafusal muscle fibres, the thin actin and the thick myosin fibres, to slide past each other, thereby shortening the overall

Table 6.1 Muscle fibre types.

Features	Type 1 Slow oxidative	Type 2a Fast oxidative	Type 2b Fast glycolytic
Metabolism	Aerobic	Aerobic and anaerobic	Anaerobic
	High in myoglobin and therefore mitochondria	High in myoglobin and mitochondria	Low in myoglobin and low in mitochondria
Amount of ATPase	Low	Intermediate	High
Twitch speed	Slow	Intermediate	Fast
Resistance to fatigue	High	Intermediate	Low
Force generated	Low	Intermediate	High
Muscle fibre diameter	Small	Large	Large
Size of anterior horn cell of motor unit	Small	Intermediate	Large

muscle length even though the filaments themselves retain their original length. The process is called excitation–contraction coupling, a term whose esoteric sophistication almost absolves the user from understanding its meaning. At present, the testing of related functions does not form part of the routine repertoire of clinical neurophysiological examination and so the reader need be burdened no further. However, should this have sparked curiosity, an additional paragraph is appended.

Muscle fibres consist of a series of in-line segments called sarcomeres. Thin actin fibres are attached to the ends of these sarcomeres at the so-called Z disc. The actin fibres do not extend over the whole length of the sarcomere. Towards its centre are thicker myosin fibres which are interleaved between the actin fibres and, like them, do not extend over the whole length of the sarcomere. When muscle contraction occurs, a series of changes takes place between them. Calcium reacts with a protein, troponin, on the actin fibre, which then causes another molecule, tropomyosin, to reveal binding sides on the actin filament. If ATP (adenosine triphosphate) is present and has been hydrolysed by the enzyme ATPase within the myosin to ADP (adenosine diphosphate) and inorganic phosphate, the energy released allows the myosin to bind to the actin, forming a so-called cross-bridge. The myosin, which is now in a high-energy state, then changes its form and pulls the actin inwards so as to shorten the length of the sarcomere. This reduces the energy state of the myosin which nevertheless remains attached to the actin. The arrival of more ATP breaks the cross-bridge connection. The process, which is repeated, is known as cross-bridge cycling. It ceases when calcium is pumped back into the sarcoplasmic reticulum, a membrane-bound calcium store within the muscle.

Some Technical Matters: Electrodes, Stimulators, Amplifiers, Display, Averagers

Electrodes

An electrode is a conductor which carries an electrical signal between two points. In the case of a stimulating electrode, the signal is carried between the stimulator output and the area close to the nerve to be stimulated. A recording electrode transmits signals from a nerve or a muscle to an amplifier.

The interface between electrode and tissue creates a barrier to the flow of current. If we were dealing with direct current, this would simply be the resistance as given by Ohm's law. But the circuits involved have time-varying as well as steady components. The opposition to current flow in these circumstances is called impedance.

All electrodes used in clinical practice are extracellular. In so-called near-nerve electrode recordings, the same electrode can also be used to stimulate the nerve. In this practice, nerve stimulation precedes recording by monitoring the stimulus strength to gauge the proximity of the electrode to the nerve. The considerable detail that recordings from this technique provide is heavily overshadowed by the fact that they require the use of needle electrodes and great skill in needle placement, and summon considerable patience and some fortitude on the part of the patient.

A recording electrode is interested in what is going on at its location. Unfortunately, to do this, like all electrodes, is it has to be part of a circuit involving a second electrode. These are called the active and reference electrodes, respectively, or the different and indifferent electrodes. The problem is that the reference or indifferent electrode is never 'indifferent'; it always registers some voltage change, often to an undesirable degree. Techniques are used to minimise this. In the case of near-nerve needle electrode recordings, the indifferent electrode is usually placed some distance away in subcutaneous tissue. Surface electrode studies of motor nerve conduction may use an active electrode over the end-plate region of the muscle and an inactive one over the tendon, the so-called belly-tendon recordings.

This also leads us to a consideration of the needle electrodes which are used in clinical practice. The skin, which keeps the water out, keeps the electricity in. At present, there is no clinically suitable alternative to a needle electrode to examine motor unit activity. The commonest variety is a concentric needle electrode in which an insulated wire is threaded down a hollow needle. Thus, at the oblique tip, there is an oval active electrode which records activity from a very small adjacent area. By contrast, the activity picked up by the reference cannula comes from a very wide area and will tend to cancel out as background noise. Needle diameters vary. Ideally, the diameter of the active recording electrode should be similar to that of the muscle or nerve fibre under scrutiny. Hence, electrodes for the examination of facial muscles are thinner than those used for limb muscles.

In order to reduce yet further the pick-up area of a needle electrode, two insulated wires can be threaded down the cannula. They become the active and reference electrodes and the cannula acts as the earth electrode, an additional connection required by most recording amplifiers. These are known as bifilar electrodes. They are seldom needed but can be invaluable when trying to record from a severely wasted muscle because activity from a different but nearby muscle will be 'seen' equally by both recording electrodes and, as discussed in the subsection 'Amplifiers', will cancel out.

In another variation, an insulated wire is brought out of a side port on the cannula. This presents a circular profile which has a smaller surface area than that of the oval one found in a standard concentric needle electrode and is therefore better suited to recording from single muscle fibres. This is the so-called single-fibre electrode used in the examination of neuromuscular function. The diameter of the housing cannula is only slightly larger than that of a standard concentric needle electrode but its manufacturing cost is considerably greater. There is now a tendency to use facial needle electrodes instead, in conjunction with adjustments to the amplifier settings, to limit the input to the high frequencies associated with the spike potentials sought.

Surface electrodes for stimulating or recording are widely used. Stimulus voltage may become high if confronted by high skin impedance, which may also increase patient discomfort. Similarly, to ensure maximum quality of signal transfer to the amplifier during recording, the impedance between the electrodes and the skin should be as low as possible. This is achieved by removing surface grease from the skin and using saline or electrode gel at the interface. Mild abrasion of the stratum corneum, which has very high electrical impedance, can be beneficial but nowadays a pumice stone is easier to use than to find.

Stimulators

It should be remembered that it is current, not voltage, that stimulates a nerve. Stimulators may be constant voltage or constant current in type, the descriptions being self-explanatory. From Ohm's law, we know that voltage equals the product of current and resistance. So a constant voltage stimulator will deliver a small and possibly insufficient current if the resistance of the tissue between the stimulator electrode and the nerve is high. Conversely, if the resistance is low, the current could, in theory, become unnecessarily excessive. A constant-current stimulator allows the stimulus strength to be directly controlled and monitored.

Amplifiers

Signals from recording electrodes are fed into a differential amplifier. This is one type of so-called operational amplifiers, or op-amps. By adorning them with different combinations of capacitors and resistors, they can perform a variety of mathematical functions, hence their name. The configuration we use is designed to amplify the differences between the inputs whilst minimising the changes common to both. In its simplest form, the amplifier is usually represented as a triangle with two inputs, a non-inverting or +ve input and an inverting or – ve input, and an output as shown in Diagram 7.1. A positive signal (say) to the non-inverting input will produce an amplified positive output. The same signal to the inverting input will create an amplified negative output.

Therefore, if the same signal is fed simultaneously to both inputs, the output of the amplifier will be zero. Or should be. This cancellation is called common mode rejection. In

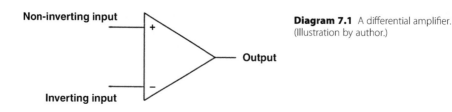

Non-inverting input

Output

Inverting input

Diagram 7.1 A differential amplifier. (Illustration by author.)

practice, rejection is never complete and so a measure called the common mode rejection ratio (CMRR) is used to quantify this shortcoming. It is expressed in decibels (dB, 20 dB = 10-fold reduction, 40 dB = 100-fold reduction, etc.) and is related to input frequency. The higher the ratio, the better. The additional benefit of a differential amplifier is that it minimises electrical interference which could otherwise overwhelm the output of the recording system.

The characteristics of this type of amplifier are exploited in the measurement of sensory and mixed nerve action potentials recorded with surface electrodes aligned along the nerve. See Chapter 8, 'Volume Conduction', for further discussion of this.

The amplifier contains controls to vary the gain (another term for amplification) of the system as well as the means to filter the passage of different frequency components in the signal. Low frequency filters allow high frequencies through, hence the alternative name high-pass filter. Similarly, with high frequency or low-pass filters. These two filters combine to allow a range of frequencies, the bandpass, to be processed by the amplifier. This facility is particularly useful in single-fibre electromyography when we are looking for spike potentials.

Amplifiers also have an audio output which can be very valuable in diagnosing spontaneous EMG activity as well as contributing towards the differentiation between myopathic and neuropathic changes. The ear is very good at pattern recognition!

Display – Oscilloscopes

The electrical signals we record are fed into an amplifier and displayed on an oscilloscope. The oscilloscope is an electronically created moving graph, from left to right of the display, which registers a vertical deflection according to the output from the amplifier. The sweep speed of the display and also the gain of the amplifier are adjusted to suit the conditions being investigated. These are shown on the screen of the EMG machine and on printouts. The gain setting appears on the display or printout as so many microvolts (µV) or millivolts (mV) per division, whilst the sweep speed is given in terms of milliseconds (ms) per division.

A free-running sweep is ideal when looking for spontaneous activity. In this case, when the sweep reaches the end of the display it restarts from the beginning. The form of the potentials and the frequency of their occurrence can be conveniently displayed.

When investigating motor unit potentials (MUPs), a so-called trigger and delay facility is invaluable. The sweep is inhibited until a potential of sufficient amplitude arrives. This then triggers the display but by means of clever electronics the whole of the potential, which is stored in a continuously updated memory, can be seen by displacing it to the right of the

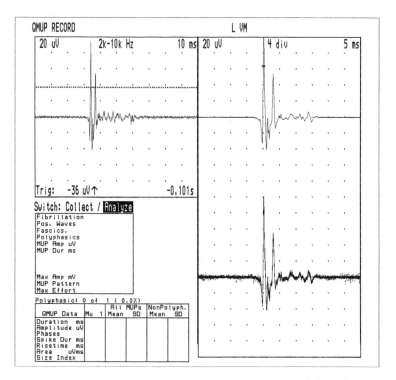

Figure 7.1 The use of trigger and delay to display a motor unit potential. (Image included with permission from the Sheffield Teaching Hospitals NHS Foundation Trust.)

sweep onset, showing what happened before the trigger point as well. This is the delay. Both the trigger level and the delay can be adjusted to facilitate inspection and measurement of the potential.

A polyphasic motor unit potential is shown in Figure 7.1. A motor unit potential is the electrical activity generated by a firing motor unit, and if it has five or more phases (i.e. crosses the baseline more than four times), it is said to be polyphasic. These topics are discussed more fully in Chapter 10, 'Electromyography (EMG)'.

When the first component exceeds the trigger level, usually shown as a dotted horizontal line as in the left window of Figure 7.1 or as a small horizontal bar as seen in the right window, the sweep is initiated. The trace on the left is displayed at a gain of 20 μV per division and a sweep speed of 10 ms per division. A potential from the same motor unit can be seen at an unchanged gain but at a faster sweep speed of 5 ms per division on the right. Potentials from repeated firings of the motor unit are superimposed below on the right. Many small, late but stable components can be clearly seen. The patient who had a history of childhood poliomyelitis presented with post-polio syndrome.

The technique is particularly useful in the investigation of neuromuscular junction abnormalities such as those seen in myasthenia gravis where unstable components of motor unit potentials are sought. It is invaluable when measuring motor unit potential duration, especially if there are small, late components.

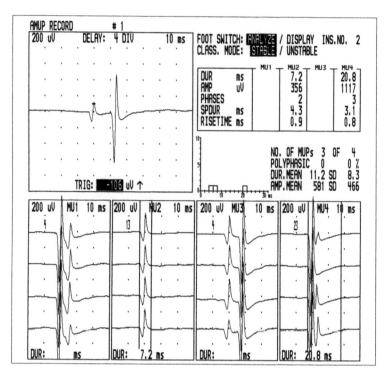

Figure 7.2 Two motor unit potentials masquerading as four. (Image included with permission from the Sheffield Teaching Hospitals NHS Foundation Trust.)

Another type of trigger and delay uses pattern recognition to help distinguish one motor unit from another, as shown in Figure 7.2. But in this example, you can see that the asynchronous firing of two motor unit potentials (one producing a relatively large signal and the other a considerably smaller one) has produced artefacts which the unwary could mistake for four separate motor unit potentials. The advantage of this technique, however, is that is allows us to study motor unit potentials of different sizes, particularly the smaller ones, which can be very helpful when looking for the characteristic small, brief potentials found in patients with a myopathy.

In nerve conduction studies, we use the sweep of the oscilloscope to help us measure the conduction time between stimulus and response. In these cases, the stimulus triggers the onset of the sweep whose speed is adjusted according to the nature of the investigation. The stimulus artefact, recorded as a result of volume conduction, can be seen at the onset of the sweep.

Averagers

Because the action potentials recorded from sensory nerves (sensory nerve action potentials or SNAPs) are normally quite small, any reduction in amplitude can cause problems and so additional recording techniques are used, which may allow otherwise undetectable potentials to be visualised. In the early days of clinical neurophysiology, a partial solution to the problem was provided by superimposing many recorded images. The potentials caused by background noise unrelated to the stimulus tended to cancel out whereas the time-locked responses were relatively prominent. Refinements of these principles have now provided us with so-called signal averagers by which sensory nerve action potentials previously too small to be visualised can now be recorded and measured. The technique increases the signal to noise ratio in proportion to the square root of the number of stimuli.

Volume Conduction

8

Intracellular recordings are one thing but apart from rare and somewhat spectacularly courageous research projects the sort of recordings we make clinically are extracellular. This means that there is some distance between the generator site and the recording electrode. We are concerned with so-called near-field potentials in which the distance is relatively small. This contrasts with far-field potentials such as evoked sensory potentials.

The detailed understanding of the ionic flows across a membrane to produce an action potential compares with the complexity of explaining how the changes are recorded and interpreted at some distance from a generator site. As every schoolkid knows, the human body is largely a bag of water containing structures, either static or moving, with varying abilities to transmit electrical charges. The transmission of an electrical potential – whether arising from intracellular activity or, more crudely, from external electrical stimulation through extracellular tissue – is called volume conduction.

Elegant but complex models have been designed to explain how the recording electrodes used in the clinic see what is happening during activity in a muscle or nerve. These include solid angle geometry looking at moving dipoles (charges of opposite polarity separated by a small distance), or considerations of the effects of source and sink currents. Fortunately, there is a simplified consensus that electrical fields moving towards, under and away from a recording electrode will produce a triphasic waveform with corresponding positive, negative and then positive components. A potential that arises directly beneath the recording electrode shows no initial positive wave; there is a negative wave corresponding to the depolarisation of the membrane followed by a positive wave caused by repolarisation. A depolarising potential that approaches the electrode but does not pass beyond it shows only a positive deflection followed by a slow restoration of the signal to its resting value. An example is the positive sharp wave, as illustrated in Chapter 10, 'Electromyography (EMG); Spontaneous EMG Activity'.

Peripheral nerves contain fibres of different diameters conducting at different speeds. At present, there is no clinically satisfactory method of comparing conduction velocities in any but the fastest conduction fibres against normal values. So how do we tell when the nerve action potentials from these fast-conducting fibres have arrived? The models of volume conduction concur that the negative peak of the triphasic potential corresponds to the moment when the active zone of depolarisation is under the electrode. But in the clinical setting, the negative peak of a nerve action potential which we record is the summation of all the negative peaks of the conducting fibres, not just the fastest ones. In near-nerve sensory recordings, the easily measurable peak of the first positive wave of the triphasic potential is calculated to approximate most closely to the arrival time of the fastest conducting fibres. Although this represents the approaching composite waveform which has not yet reached

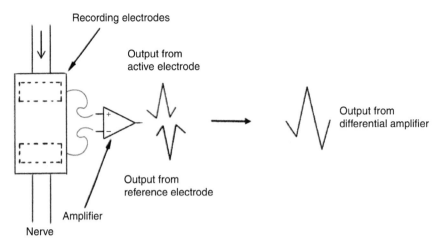

Recording electrodes

Output from
active electrode

Output from
differential amplifier

Output from
reference electrode

Amplifier

Nerve

Diagram 8.1 Volume-conducted triphasic potentials can augment each other. (Illustration by author.)

the recording electrode, the potential from those which arrived first has been obscured. Life is full of compromises; this may not be the worst.

In an EMG clinic, sensory and mixed nerve action potentials are usually recorded with surface electrodes aligned along the nerve as shown in Diagram 8.1. The potentials are, at best, quite small because of the attenuating effect of the distance between source and electrode and also because of the impedance barrier of the skin. The recording arrangement offers the possibility of some amplification through summation. Both electrodes will record a triphasic potential but, when connected to a differential amplifier, these will be of opposite polarity.

Consider the triphasic action potential recorded by the active electrode. Shortly afterwards, the same potential is recorded by the reference electrode. As we have seen in Chapter 7, 'Some Technical Matters; Amplifiers', the same voltage at each amplifier input registers an upward deflection when presented to one and a downward when presented to the other. So the triphasic potential recorded by the reference electrode is inverted. Because the time interval between the two is very short, when they are summed the phases tend to reinforce one another, resulting in an augmented nerve action potential. This effect could be lost if there is slowed conduction. It will definitely be lost if the inter-electrode distance is too long, which is why recording electrode configurations should be standardised in each clinic.

In the case of sensory nerve action potentials, there are a number of reproducible points which can be selected to estimate the conduction time in the fastest fibres. These include the first positive peak, the point at which the rising phase of the negatively moving potential crosses the baseline and the negative peak itself. Clinical reports should clearly state what measurements have been made.

As mentioned, when the volume-conducted potential arises beneath the recording electrode, only a negative–positive diphasic potential will be recorded. This of importance in motor conduction studies. If the recording electrode is over the end-plate region, the first deflection will be negative. If, however, it is distant from the end-plate region, there will be an initial positive wave. The measurement of conduction time from stimulus to muscle becomes problematic. Furthermore, the badly positioned recording electrode will record a smaller-than-normal peak amplitude, which could be erroneously interpreted as a loss of nerve or muscle fibre. An alternative explanation of an initial positive wave is that it is arising from a response in a different muscle. This should alert the examiner to the possibility of unwanted spread of stimulus current to a nerve other than the one under investigation.

Chapter 9

Pathology

Muscle

Whilst all muscle fibre types may be vulnerable in some disorders such as polymyositis, selective involvement of specific types of muscle fibre is seen, for example, in steroid myopathy which affects type 2 fibres. This is important because type 1 fibres which generate low force are the first to be recruited in the sort of moderate contraction called for when assessing motor unit potentials. By the time type 2 fibres are recruited, the amount of EMG activity is so great that it becomes impossible to analyse individual different motor units.

The distribution of myopathic change varies according to the type and degree of pathology. The selection of the muscle or muscles to be examined will clearly be determined by the clinical features. It should be understood that myopathy tends to be a patchy disorder which may yield false negative results. Also, mild involvement of a muscle can easily be missed whereas severe change leaves very little muscle tissue yielding characteristic EMG abnormality. The three bears and their porridge spring to mind. It also reminds us that the practice of electromyography is often known as 'sampling'.

Nerve

As noted in Chapter 2, 'Basic Anatomy and a Little Physiology', the peripheral nerve axon is an elongated extension of the cell body. In some cases, it may be ensheathed in segments of myelin produced by the Schwann cells.

Given these two main components of peripheral nerves, it follows that there are two main categories of pathology: degeneration, also known as axonal degeneration, and demyelination, as depicted in Diagram 9.1.

Demyelination occurs when there is pathology affecting the Schwann cells. This may occur as a result of local pathology as in compression neuropathy or as part of a more widespread disorder as in peripheral neuropathy. Patchy involvement of Schwann cells is characteristic of demyelinating peripheral neuropathy, hence the descriptive term 'segmental demyelination'.

Depending on the degree of pathology, nerve conduction across a demyelinated region is either slowed or blocked. If demyelination is severe, it evolves to degeneration. The effects of these changes are detailed in Chapter 14, 'Nerve Conduction Studies: Demyelination'.

Sufficiently severe trauma to a nerve causes degeneration distal to the lesion, so-called Wallerian degeneration. Degeneration may take several days to occur and so there is a period when normal nerve conduction findings will belie the gravity of the situation – a trap for the unwary.

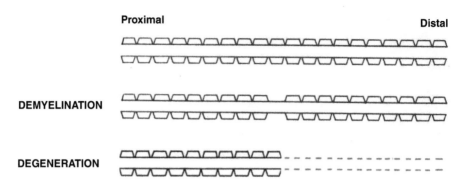

Proximal   **Distal**

DEMYELINATION

DEGENERATION

Diagram 9.1 The different types of pathology affecting myelinated peripheral nerves. (Image included with permission from the Sheffield Teaching Hospitals NHS Foundation Trust.)

Degeneration also occurs in some types of peripheral neuropathy. The cell body of the axon transports material essential to the health of the peripheral nerve along its whole extent. This is quite some undertaking. If pathology strikes the cell body, it is not surprising that the effects are felt first at the extremities of the nerve. The changes are most marked in the longest nerves. Progressive disease causes centripetal change in the nerve, hence the term 'dying-back neuropathy'. Nerve conduction studies may show a reduction in the amplitudes of sensory nerve action potentials and, in severe cases, those of the compound muscle action potentials as well. A compound muscle action potential is the summation of all the action potentials from muscle fibres activated by stimulation of their nerve supply. Nerve conduction velocities are either normal or show a slight reduction corresponding to the degeneration of the largest diameter, that is, the fastest conducting, fibres. Chapter 13, 'Nerve Conduction Studies: Degeneration', describes these matters in more detail.

On electromyography, spontaneous activity such as fibrillation potentials and positive sharp waves may be seen. These arise from single muscle fibres that have lost their nerve supply. The electrical activity recorded from a muscle during maximal voluntary effort is called the recruitment pattern. It becomes reduced if some motor units have lost their nerve supply and so become unable to contribute to it. Peripheral nerves have great capacity for regeneration, although not always to a clinically beneficial extent. In the process, they produce motor unit potentials of increased duration which aid diagnosis. All these changes are described in Chapter 10, 'Electromyography (EMG)'.

Electromyography (EMG)

Electromyography is the study of electrical potentials recorded from muscles. It is used to differentiate primary muscle disease (myopathy) from abnormalities within the muscle resulting from pathology of its nerve supply (neuropathy). The fine diagnostic detail required necessitates the use of a concentric needle electrode, which limits its patient appeal. The examiner aims to obtain a representative selection of motor unit activity and to detect any spontaneously occurring activity.

In myopathy, muscle fibres are lost from many motor units which therefore become smaller, the size of the motor unit being proportional to the number of muscle fibres it contains, as described in Chapter 2, 'Basic Anatomy and a Little Physiology; Motor System'. Motor unit numbers, however, remain normal until a late stage in the process when all the muscle fibres from one or more motor units have been lost. It is notable that, in many cases, the muscle fibres are also abnormally soft, imparting a 'myopathic consistency' to the exploring electrode.

Pathology within the peripheral nerve may target the axon or its myelin. Demyelinating neuropathies alter nerve conduction velocities and will be considered in Chapter 14, 'Nerve Conduction Studies: Demyelination'. Axonal pathology leads to degeneration of the nerve. The muscle fibres which lose their nerve supply as a result, tend to attract new growth from the nearby nerve terminals of an adjacent nerve fibre. The process is called collateral re-innervation, regeneration or 'sprouting'. All this leads to two changes. First, the number of motor units within the muscle becomes smaller. But the motor units that have incorporated the previously denervated muscle fibres become larger.

Myopathy and Neuropathy

To distinguish the pathologies of myopathy and neuropathy, we need to be able to measure the number of motor units and their size.

Motor Unit Size

During voluntary muscle contraction, the potentials resulting from the activity of each muscle fibre within the motor unit, the muscle action potentials, summate to form a motor unit potential (MUP), also known as a motor unit action potential (MUAP). The amplitude of the MUP is clearly proportional to the number of its constituent muscle action potentials. Unfortunately, the beguiling option of measuring MUP amplitude and thus assessing motor unit size is severely constrained by technical factors because the amplitude declines exponentially as the distance from the generator

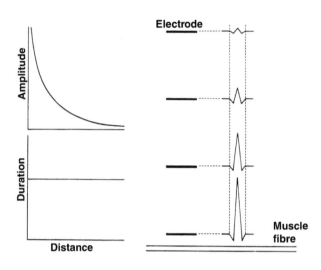

Diagram 10.1 The effect of electrode distance from the generator site on the amplitude and duration of the recorded potential. (Image included with permission from the Sheffield Teaching Hospitals NHS Foundation Trust.)

site to the recording electrode increases. Fortunately, there is an indirect measure of motor unit size, the key to which is contained in Diagram 10.1.

Although the MUP amplitude changes dramatically with changes in the position of the recording electrode, the MUP duration does not. The MUP duration is the time interval between the departure of the potential from the baseline to its final return. As we will now see, this can be used as an indirect method of assessing motor unit size.

The nerve terminals to a muscle are distributed over a relatively short segment called the end-plate region, or end-plate zone, located at its mid-point. A nerve action potential arriving at a muscle depolarises all the end-plates at virtually the same time. The muscle action potentials then propagate to either end of the muscle at a fairly constant and relatively slow speed of about 4 m/s.

In Diagram 10.2, inset (a) shows how a nerve action potential is propagated from the end-plate towards the ends of the muscle fibre.

In (b) we see a couple of muscle fibres with a concentric needle electrode inserted to one side of the end-plate zone. Because the muscle action potentials arrive at different times at the recording electrode, reflecting the differences in the length of their conduction paths along the muscle, the duration of the resultant MUP is greater than that of the individual muscle action potentials which comprise it. The asynchronous arrival of these muscle action potentials is called temporal dispersion. The duration of the MUP is therefore proportional to the scatter or spatial dispersion of the end-plates.

In neuropathy, the newly formed end-plates resulting from collateral re-innervation tend to extend over a greater area than the end-plate zone of the donor motor unit. This increased spatial dispersion of the end-plates leads to increased temporal dispersion of the MUP and hence an increase in its duration.

To aid clarity, the following two diagrams show the end-plates from only a few muscle fibres in the motor unit. In Diagram 10.3, after the nerve in motor unit **B** degenerates,

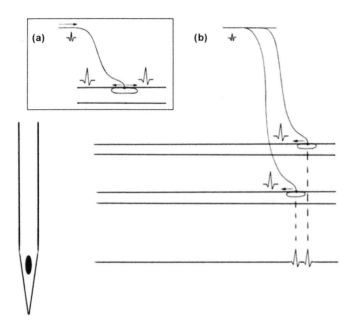

Diagram 10.2a Muscle action potentials travel in both directions from the end-plate. (Illustration by author.)

Diagram 10.2b The duration of the motor unit potential is proportional to the spatial scatter of the end-plates. (Illustration by author.)

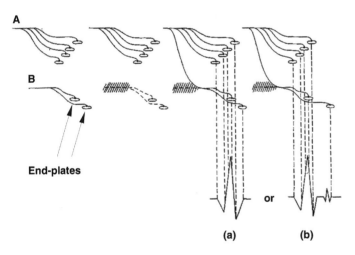

Diagram 10.3 The increase in motor unit potential duration due to collateral re-innervation (a) which may produce a satellite potential (b). (Image included with permission from the Sheffield Teaching Hospitals NHS Foundation Trust.)

collateral re-innervation from motor unit **A** leads to an increase in the spatial scatter of the end-plates of this donor motor unit.

Sometimes, a very late component of the MUP is seen, a so-called satellite potential. This is due either to the extreme location of the relevant end-plate, or to slowed conduction in an immature regenerating nerve fibre, or both.

Figure 10.1 shows an example of this in the free-running display where some normal-duration MUPs are seen together with one of increased duration which also bears a satellite potential, denoted by the asterisk.

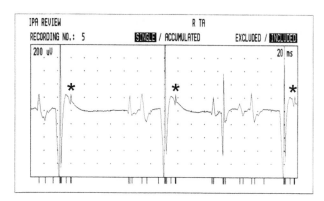

Figure 10.1 A motor unit potential of increased duration incorporating a satellite potential denoted by the asterisk. (Image included with permission from the Sheffield Teaching Hospitals NHS Foundation Trust.)

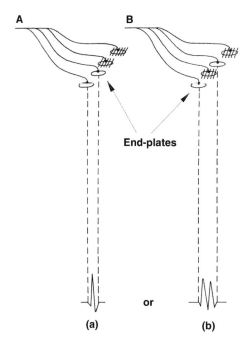

Diagram 10.4 The reduction in motor unit potential duration due to loss of muscle fibres (a) which may produce polyphasia (b). (Image included with permission from the Sheffield Teaching Hospitals NHS Foundation Trust.)

In myopathy, muscle fibres are lost in a patchy distribution which, sooner or later, leads to a reduction in the length of the end-plate zone. The reduced spatial dispersion of the end-plates causes reduced temporal dispersion of the individual muscle action potentials and therefore an MUP of shorter-than-normal duration. This is shown in Diagram 10.4.

In Figure 10.2, we see examples of normal (**A**), myopathic (**B**) and neuropathic (**C**) MUPs showing normal, reduced and increased durations, respectively. Individual MUPs

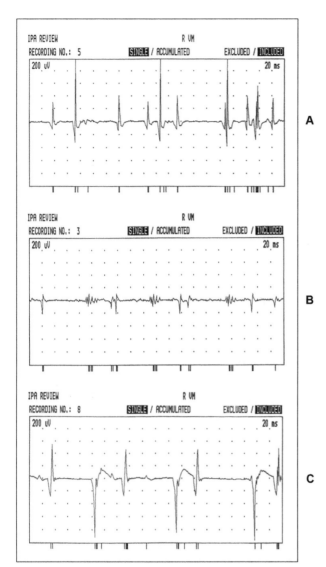

Figure 10.2 Examples of motor unit potentials recorded from a normal muscle (**A**), a myopathy (**B**) and a neuropathy (**C**). (Image included with permission from the Sheffield Teaching Hospitals NHS Foundation Trust.)

can be clearly distinguished on these free-running displays but, in cases of difficulty, trigger and delay facilities are often helpful.

So far, we have concentrated on the duration of the MUP. Electrical potentials have three distinctive characteristics: amplitude, duration and form. We have seen that amplitude is an unreliable guide to motor unit size except in extreme forms of pathology when MUPs are smaller than normal in myopathy and larger than normal in neuropathy. We have also noted that the duration of the MUP, which is determined by the longitudinal distribution (spatial scatter) of the motor unit end-plates, is

Table 10.1 Motor unit potentials in neuropathy and myopathy.

Motor unit potential	Neuropathy	Myopathy
Duration	Increased	Reduced
Amplitude	(Increased)	(Reduced)
Form	Polyphasic	Polyphasic

decreased in myopathy and increased in neuropathy. In both types of pathology, the distribution of end-plates within the end-plate region tends to become somewhat uneven as a result of additional outlying end-plates in neuropathy and drop-out of end-plates in myopathy. This leads, in both cases, to a rather disorderly arrival of muscle action potentials at the recording electrode and thus to an increase in the number of peaks and troughs of the MUP as shown in Diagrams 10.3 and 10.4. Potentials which have five or more phases (or peaks) are called polyphasic. Excessive numbers of polyphasic potentials (more than 15%) represent pathology but do not distinguish which type.

Table 10.1 summarises the motor unit potential changes found in neuropathy and myopathy.

Because MUP amplitude tends to be greater in neuropathy and smaller in myopathy, the amplitude of the segment of the potential recorded between the 'turns' (i.e. changes in phase or direction) of a MUP will follow a similar trend. This concept has been incorporated into semi-automatic turns-amplitude analysers. The method requires careful attention to technique but in skilled hands has been shown to be useful, particularly in the detection of myopathy.

The sound generated by an EMG signal can often be of diagnostic help. The myopathic potentials of brief duration tend to give a high-pitched sound contrasting with the low-pitched one associated with the long duration potentials of neuropathic disorders.

A Note on EMG Technique

In concentric needle electrode studies of normal muscle, the spike component of a MUP arises from about 5 to 10 muscle fibres within 1 mm of the recording surface. Motor units differ greatly in size from small, in facial muscles, to large, in thigh muscles. Muscles which are commonly examined in the clinic probably have motor units containing 200 to 300 muscle fibres arranged fairly uniformly in a cylindrical fashion alongside other motor units, with some of which they intermingle.

After a needle is inserted into a muscle, details of motor unit activity are registered. The needle is then withdrawn slightly. Depending on the degree of withdrawal, the same motor unit or units may still be recorded but their shape will change corresponding to the relationship between conduction distance and amplitude described earlier. If the withdrawal is gradual and attention is paid to motor unit firing frequency and MUP duration, it is usually possible to identify if and when a new MUP is picked up.

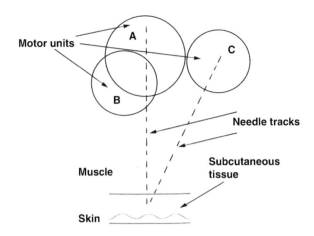

Diagram 10.5 A method to avoid repeated sampling of the same motor unit. (Illustration by author.)

To avoid repeated recording from the same motor units, the needle can either be re-inserted (involving another skin puncture) or withdrawn into the subcutaneous tissue and then re-introduced into the muscle along a different plane. Diagram 10.5 illustrates this technique showing how activity from motor unit C can be recorded.

The method does not, however, absolve the examiner from the need to make repeated insertions when, for example, hunting mild neuropathic change or an elusive myopathy.

Motor Unit Numbers

The strength of a muscle contraction is proportional to two factors. First, the number of motor units recruited and second, their firing frequency. At the onset of voluntary contraction the concentric needle electrode will often pick up only one MUP. As the subject increases the strength of voluntary contraction two things happen. First, the motor unit that is firing increases its firing rate and second, the number of motor units recruited also increases. These processes continue pari passu with the force of contraction. The recorded potentials form what is known as a recruitment pattern as shown in Diagram 10.6.

At maximal voluntary effort in a normal muscle, individual potentials become merged and so cannot be separately identified. This is sometimes called an interference pattern.

If the number of motor units in a muscle is significantly reduced, an interference pattern will not be realised. Instead, the pattern will be correspondingly sparse. This reduced pattern will, if severe, allow individual motor units to be identified, a so-called pattern of discrete activity. We look for a reduced pattern to diagnose loss of motor units and therefore neuropathy. In myopathy, where motor units are smaller than normal because muscle fibres have been lost, recruitment of additional motor units compensates for this and may lead to the seemingly paradoxical situation in which submaximal voluntary effort generates a full interference pattern.

Figure 10.3 shows an example of a full interference pattern.

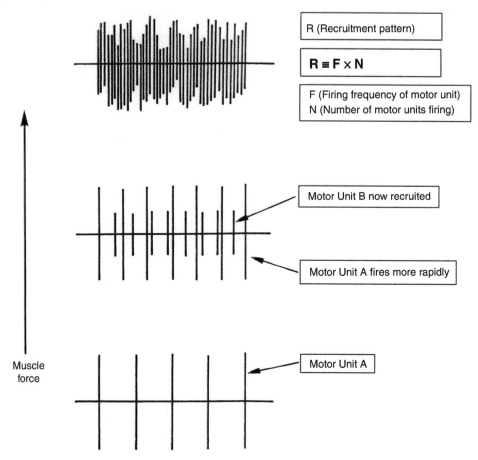

R (Recruitment pattern)

$$R \equiv F \times N$$

F (Firing frequency of motor unit)
N (Number of motor units firing)

Motor Unit B now recruited

Motor Unit A fires more rapidly

Motor Unit A

Muscle force

Diagram 10.6 The recruitment pattern is proportional to the number of motor units firing and their firing frequency. (Image included with permission from the Sheffield Teaching Hospitals NHS Foundation Trust.)

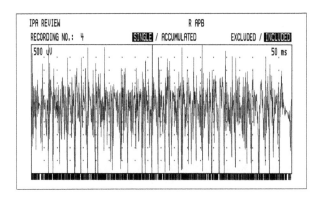

Figure 10.3 A normal recruitment pattern, sometimes called a full interference pattern. (Image included with permission from the Sheffield Teaching Hospitals NHS Foundation Trust.)

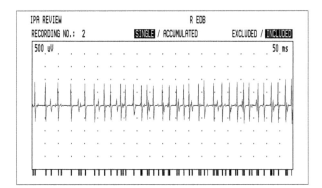

Figure 10.4 A markedly reduced recruitment pattern, sometimes called a pattern of discrete activity. (Image included with permission from the Sheffield Teaching Hospitals NHS Foundation Trust.)

This contrasts with Figure 10.4, which depicts an example of a markedly reduced pattern, a pattern of discrete activity.

To this straightforward clinical application of basic neurophysiology we now have to admit to two major drawbacks. The first and rather surprising one is that there is currently no satisfactory objective method of measuring the density of the recruitment pattern from which the number of active motor units may be inferred. The second and less surprising one concerns the effect of the concentric needle electrode itself. Although muscle is primarily concerned with motor function, it does contain some sensory nerves which relay a feeling of deep pressure and some discomfort at the tip of the needle. Most patients tolerate this very well and provide powerful contractions. Nevertheless, all this leads to two subjective estimates: the degree of voluntary contraction and the density of the recruitment pattern.

In moderate to severe cases of neuropathy where the pattern is markedly reduced in the context of good voluntary effort, the technique is clinically valuable. In others, where there is uncertainty about the degree of voluntary effort and no more than a questionable, border-line reduction in the density of the recruitment pattern, less so. The recruitment pattern is usually normal in myopathy but in severe, end-stage cases all muscle fibres from individual motor units may be lost, resulting in reduced numbers of motor units and therefore a reduced recruitment pattern.

Spontaneous EMG Activity

So far, we have been considering what happens when we record EMG activity during voluntary effort. Sometimes activity is recorded when the muscle is at rest.

When a needle is inserted into a muscle, there is a brief electrical discharge as a result of the mechanical excitation of muscle fibres. This is called insertional activity. Unsuccessful attempts have been made to show that its duration, which tends to be increased in pathology, can be clinically useful.

If the needle is inserted into a muscle at or very close to the end-plate region, the normally occurring miniature end-plate potentials, as described in Chapter 5, 'The Neuromuscular Junction', are picked up as excessive background noise, **end-plate noise**. There may also be some from the patient since this part of the muscle is relatively tender.

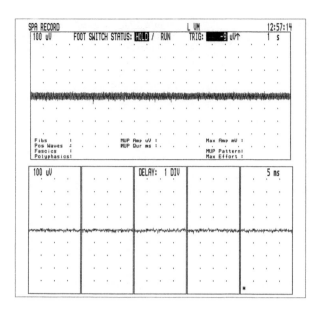

Figure 10.5 End-plate noise. (Image included with permission from the Sheffield Teaching Hospitals NHS Foundation Trust.)

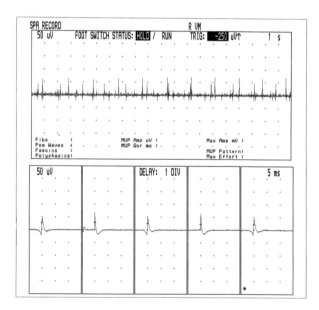

Figure 10.6 End-plate potentials. (Image included with permission from the Sheffield Teaching Hospitals NHS Foundation Trust.)

The free-running traces in Figure 10.5 show this noise at different sweep speeds.

Sometimes an **end-plate potential** itself may be seen, identified as a biphasic potential, as in Figure 10.6. Its initial negative phase indicates that it has arisen locally. Its duration is 5 ms or less and it fires irregularly. It represents the summation of miniature end-plate

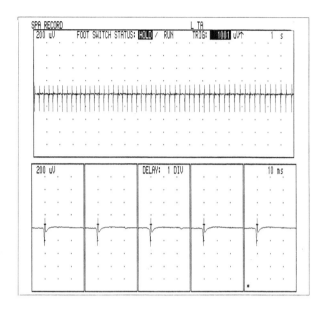

Figure 10.7 Fibrillation potentials. (Image included with permission from the Sheffield Teaching Hospitals NHS Foundation Trust.)

potentials sufficient in numbers to produce it but insufficient to generate a propagated muscle action potential.

In this figure and similar screenshots where 'DELAY' appears in the lower section, trigger and delay facilities have been used. The duration of the delay is given and a small horizontal mark denotes the trigger level. Compared with the upper trace, the sweep speed has been increased but the gain remains unchanged. In this way, the free-running upper trace shows the firing pattern whilst the lower section displays the duration, amplitude and form of the potentials.

In this example, the free-running trace shows low voltage background noise with some larger, irregularly firing potentials. The lower section shows that some of these are typical diphasic end-plate potentials of 5 ms duration or less. There are also some similar potentials but with an initial positive phase. These are also end-plate potentials which are originating a little way from the recording electrode and picked up by volume conduction.

Fibrillation potentials, shown in Figure 10.7, usually denote neuropathy. Less frequently, they may be seen in some myopathies such as polymyositis, although in these cases the question of a co-existent but subordinate neuropathy has been raised. The potentials are triphasic, of 5 ms or less duration, and may continue to fire for many seconds, usually at a fairly regular rate of about 10 Hz or less, before tapering off. They create a distinctive sound in the loudspeaker of the recording system akin to that of frying bacon. It is thought that they arise because, after denervation, acetylcholine receptors, which are normally restricted to the end-plate zone, become widely distributed over the length of the muscle fibre making it more susceptible to depolarisation. They tend to be profuse immediately after acute lesions, much less so in chronic pathology. In this case, the sweep speed in the lower window has been reduced to 10 ms.

Positive sharp waves are thought to be fibrillation potentials occurring in a damaged muscle fibre. In this case, the depolarisation wave, which travels towards but not beyond the recording electrode, shows only the first positive component of the triphasic wave. There is then a slow decline, usually over 10–30 ms, to the resting state. Positive sharp waves which are frequently recorded together with fibrillation potentials carry the same clinical significance.

An example of positive sharp waves is shown in Figure 10.8.

Fasciculation potentials are spontaneously occurring MUPs. They are said to arise in the distal part of the motor axon and are most often but not exclusively associated with motor neurone disease. If they are not visible clinically, detection by palpation may offer the prospect of a successful recording site. As a rule, more than one potential occurs – sometimes repeated, sometimes not.

Typical fasciculation potentials are shown in Figure 10.9. Their firing rate is irregular and commonly very infrequent, often necessitating considerable patience to capture them. The lower section demonstrates that there are at least three different MUPs involved.

Fasciculation can easily be distinguished from **incomplete relaxation** in which normally occurring MUPs are recruited in a fixed, reproducible sequence. In Figure 10.10, we see that the same motor unit fires before and after a period of inactivity.

So-called benign fasciculation potentials can sometimes be shown to be driven voluntarily and differ from the pathological variety in being free from association with muscle weakness, wasting, reflex abnormality or other EMG changes.

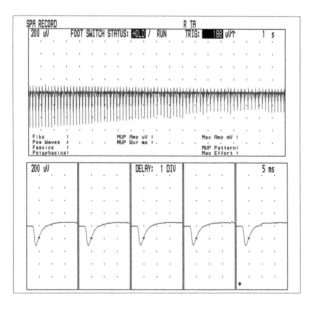

Figure 10.8 Positive sharp waves. (Image included with permission from the Sheffield Teaching Hospitals NHS Foundation Trust.)

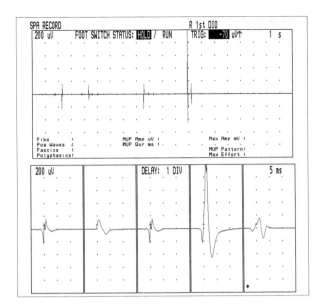

Figure 10.9 Fasciculation potentials. (Image included with permission from the Sheffield Teaching Hospitals NHS Foundation Trust.)

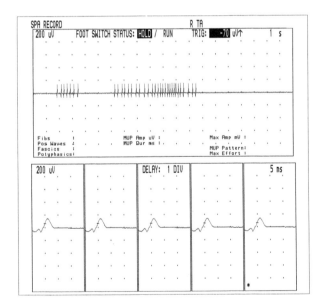

Figure 10.10 Incomplete relaxation. (Image included with permission from the Sheffield Teaching Hospitals NHS Foundation Trust.)

Myotonia is one of the most distinctive of the spontaneously occurring EMG potentials. It may be provoked by tapping the muscle or slight movement of the needle electrode. The traditional descriptive term of a 'dive bomber sound' is probably and thankfully lost on current practitioners of electromyography. But if their imagination

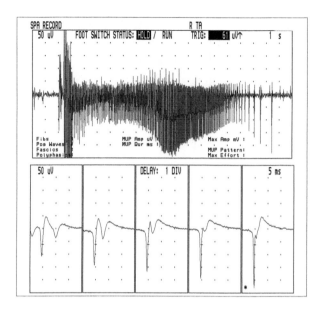

Figure 10.11 Myotonia. (Image included with permission from the Sheffield Teaching Hospitals NHS Foundation Trust.)

cannot meet the challenge, comparison with the sound of a flamboyantly driven motor cycle may suffice. The discharge, which contains potentials that often look similar to positive sharp waves repeating with an unmistakeable waxing and waning of amplitude and frequency, usually trails off but can end fairly abruptly, as in Figure 10.11. It is found mainly but not exclusively in myotonic disorders such as dystrophia myotonica and thought to be related to changes in sodium and/or calcium conductance leading to increased membrane excitability. The phenomenon may also be induced or exacerbated by cold.

In **myokymia**, grouped discharges looking like clustered MUPs repeat at regular or fairly regular intervals ranging from about 1 Hz or less to 10 Hz. The clusters may contain doublets, triplets or other multiples of these potentials, usually in varying combinations over time. The steady firing rate resembles the sound of marching. Discharges tend to be very prolonged.

In Figure 10.12, we see an example of myokymia with a typical firing pattern.

Figure 10.13, displays a section of this free-running trace at a faster sweep speed to demonstrate the mainly 'triplet' character of the discharges.

A number of lower motor neurone abnormalities have been associated with it as has, interestingly, multiple sclerosis affecting facial muscles. Clinical evidence of myokymia, namely the worm-like undulations of the affected muscle, may be seen at the same time when the face is involved but is rarely visible in the limbs unless the patient has neuromyotonia. Among postulated causes is the ephaptic, or side to side, transmission in demyelinated nerves.

Complex repetitive discharges, shown in Figure 10.14 and formerly called pseudomyotonic discharges, are characterised by the abrupt onset and cessation of a simple or complex waveform firing at a fairly constant and rapid rate. They are thought to arise from ephaptic

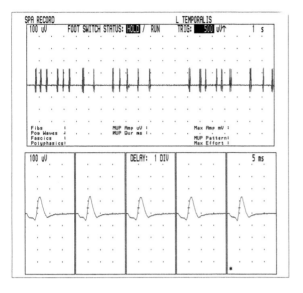

Figure 10.12 Myokymia recorded at a slow sweep speed showing the 'marching' pattern of the discharge. (Image included with permission from the Sheffield Teaching Hospitals NHS Foundation Trust.)

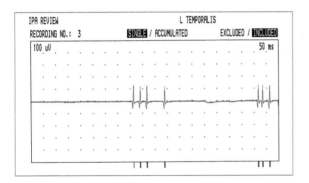

Figure 10.13 Myokymia recorded at a faster sweep speed showing the 'triplets'. (Image included with permission from the Sheffield Teaching Hospitals NHS Foundation Trust.)

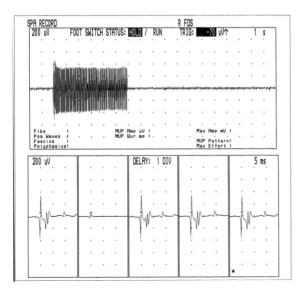

Figure 10.14 Complex repetitive discharges. (Image included with permission from the Sheffield Teaching Hospitals NHS Foundation Trust.)

transmission between muscle fibres. They are rare but said to be evidence of either myopathic or neuropathic disease.

Although EMG is invaluable in helping to diagnose a myopathy it can provide very little additional useful information unless myotonia is also found. Further refinement of the diagnosis will require additional resources such as muscle biopsy, metabolic studies and genetic information.

If EMG discloses the presence of neuropathic change, continued electrophysiological examination using nerve conduction studies will often clarify the diagnosis.

Nerve Conduction Studies (NCS): Introduction

Most peripheral nerves are mixed nerves, that is to say they contain sensory and motor fibres. If we stimulate a mixed nerve, the action potential recorded further along the nerve is called a nerve action potential or, more usually, a mixed nerve action potential (MNAP). This can be helpful but since neurological conditions may affect sensory and motor nerves differently, it is important to be able to test them separately. Diagram 11.1 shows the principle of the approach used.

In the case of motor nerves, we simply stimulate a mixed nerve and record from a muscle. The recorded response is called a compound muscle action potential (CMAP) because it represents the sum of all the muscle action potentials within the muscle that have been activated. It is noteworthy that because a single motor nerve fibre innervates many muscle fibres, Mother Nature provides an inbuilt amplifier effect, making CMAPs much easier to record than nerve action potentials.

Sensory nerves pose more of a challenge. In the upper limb, the motor components within the median and ulnar nerves to the intrinsic hand muscles terminate there but the sensory components extend to the tips of the digits. So, by stimulating digital nerves and recording over a mixed nerve, we can measure sensory conduction. In this case, the response is called the sensory action potential (SAP) or sensory nerve action potential (SNAP). In theory, the same advantages are offered in the feet, but technical factors associated with satisfactory electrode placement make this an option which is rarely used. When we stimulate a sensory

MOTOR

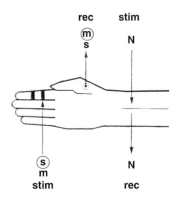

Diagram 11.1 Principles underlying the independent examination of motor and sensory nerves. (Image included with permission from the Sheffield Teaching Hospitals NHS Foundation Trust.)

SENSORY

nerve distally and record proximally, this is called orthodromic conduction since the direction of travel of the potential is the same as that of the normally transmitted impulses.

Another method for trying to measure sensory conduction is to stimulate a mixed nerve but record only from its sensory fibres. For example, the median or ulnar nerve is stimulated at the wrist and potentials recorded from the digital sensory nerves. In this case, the potential travels in the opposite direction to normal, physiologically transmitted sensory impulses and is called antidromic conduction. The unavoidable stimulation of the motor nerves produces an unwanted CMAP artefact, which can interfere with the clear identification of the sensory potential being sought.

Sensory nerve conduction is also measured if we choose a branch of a peripheral nerve which contains only sensory nerve fibres, such as the sural nerve at the ankle or the sensory branch of the radial nerve in the forearm.

Stimulation

Some patients are understandably anxious about the notion of electrical stimulation, fearing that they are about to be connected direct to the National Grid. It should be remembered though that peripheral nerve stimulation may, by definition, be imperceptible, as in sub-threshold stimulation.

As we have seen in Chapter 3, 'Peripheral Nerve: Types', peripheral nerves are composed of three main subgroups: large-diameter myelinated fibres, small-diameter myelinated fibres and unmyelinated fibres. The aim is to use a stimulus strength which is just sufficient to stimulate all the fibres in the first two groups. It is achieved by noting the size of the evoked SNAP, MNAP or CMAP as the stimulus strength is slowly increased, and then making a very small increase in the stimulus strength once these amplitudes cease to grow. This is a so-called just supramaximal stimulus, hereafter called a supramaximal stimulus. Further increases in stimulus strength are both pointless and counterproductive since they begin to activate the unmyelinated fibres from which potentials are generally too small to record and, more particularly, which also carry pain fibres. The use of ratios to calculate the strength of the supramaximal stimulus relative to the threshold stimulus are extremely unreliable and should be discouraged.

Loss of axons will cause a reduction in the number of action potentials conveyed along individual nerve fibres and therefore a reduction in the amplitude of the SNAP, MNAP or CMAP. Loss of myelin causes slowing of nerve conduction. Because there is no reliable method of measuring conduction velocities in any of the peripheral nerve fibres other than the largest diameter ones, when we compare a patient's result with a normal database, we need to be sure we are comparing like with like. In other words, we need to be sure that we have stimulated the largest diameter fibres. It might be argued that since the largest diameter fibres have the lowest stimulus threshold, this level of stimulation should suffice. However, the stimulating current must negotiate a pathway to the nerve which contains elements of mixed and sometimes high impedance. So, a supramaximal stimulus ensures that the largest diameter fibres have been stimulated and also all the myelinated fibres which contribute to the amplitude of the SNAP, MNAP or CMAP.

Factors Influencing Nerve Conduction

Nerve conduction is an energy-dependent process. Low temperature will reduce the rate of the dependent metabolic processes and so cause a reduction in conduction velocity. It is therefore very important to ensure that limbs are not cold when performing nerve conduction measurements. This is especially relevant when examining the extremities; for example, when measuring SNAPs at the wrist or ankle.

We have also seen that conduction velocity depends on the internal flow of sodium ions along the axon. Nerves taper distally and so conduction velocity over these segments is slower than over proximal ones. Curiously, although peripheral nerves in the leg are generally of larger diameter than those in the arm, the conduction velocities are slower. Differences in distal temperatures have been cited, as have 'conversion factors', but the author is unaware of a satisfactory explanation.

Conduction velocities also vary with age. They do not reach the values of mature nerves until about three to five years of age. Later in life, the modest decline which one might anticipate consonant with advancing age is seen. There is also a reduction in the size of nerve action potentials corresponding to axonal degeneration.

Other factors which have been correlated with nerve conduction velocity include gender, race, height and body mass index. The essential point is that each clinic should standardise its methods of examination and its interpretation of results.

Younger patients often like to have an appreciation of their own conduction velocities in more everyday terms. So, a conduction velocity of 50 m/s is approximately 110 mph. This is, of course, very different from electrical transmission rates of about 300 million m/s or 670 million mph, the difference being due to the distinction between ionic and electronic conduction.

Chapter 12

Nerve Conduction Studies: Normal

Normal Sensory and Mixed Nerve Conduction Studies

Sensory nerve studies are used much more frequently than mixed nerve studies. The principles of stimulation, recording and interpretation are the same for both and so for the remainder of the discussion we shall refer only to the sensory type.

Sensory nerve conduction studies provide us with two main measurements: sensory conduction velocity (SCV) and the amplitude of the sensory nerve action potential (SNAP). The form of the potential is an additional, important but less objective component.

The SCV is obtained quite simply by dividing the sensory conduction time from stimulus to recorded response into the conduction distance between the stimulating and recording electrodes, as shown in Diagram 12.1.

Because of volume conduction, the stimulus artefact, being an electromagnetic impulse, is instantaneous. This triggers the sweep of the display. The precise moment that the action potentials begin to pass beneath the active recording electrode must be estimated. The best estimate is obtained using the first positive peak of the triphasic potential, as described in Chapter 8, 'Volume Conduction'. Careful attention to technique should ensure that stimulus artefact does not obscure or deform it. In all conduction studies, sensory or motor, the cathode of the stimulator, not the anode, should be closer to the recording electrodes and, similarly, the active electrode, not the reference electrode, should be closer to the stimulator. The conduction distance is measured from the stimulating cathode to the active recording electrode. Providing the stimulus is supramaximal, the SCV represents conduction velocity in the largest diameter, fastest conducting fibres.

The SNAP amplitude is proportional to the number of fibres conducting and an important measurement, especially when investigating degenerative neuropathy. It is usually measured from the first positive peak to the negative peak or from the negative peak to the second positive peak. It goes without saying that the method chosen should be consistent.

The amplitude of a nerve action potential is not only adversely affected by the impedance of structures between the nerve and the recording electrode but also exponentially by the distance involved. These can be significant factors when the skin is dry and/or thick and, for example, when trying to record over relatively proximal sites in obese patients.

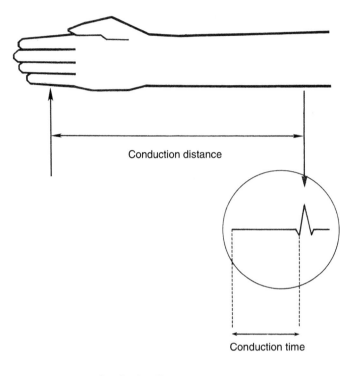

Diagram 12.1 Measurement of sensory conduction velocity. (Image included with permission from the Sheffield Teaching Hospitals NHS Foundation Trust.)

Conduction distance

Conduction time

$$\frac{\text{Conduction distance}}{\text{Conduction time}} = \text{Conduction velocity} \left(\text{SCV}\right)$$

Normal Motor Conduction Studies

In order to examine conduction in motor nerves, we simply record from a muscle supplied by the nerve. The recording electrode may be a needle or surface electrode. If a needle electrode has already been used for an EMG examination, it becomes a simple matter to continue with a motor nerve conduction study.

Because the motor nerve axon terminates at a neuromuscular junction, the analysis of motor nerve conduction provides us with two measurements, the motor conduction velocity (MCV) and the distal latency.

In normal subjects, the conduction time from, say, the elbow to the wrist is only slightly longer than the conduction time from the wrist to the muscle innervated by the nerve. This is because as the nerve approaches the muscle, it tapers, causing conduction velocity to slow (see Chapter 4, 'Peripheral Nerve Function') and, even more significantly, its terminals are no longer myelinated. So, the fast saltatory conduction now becomes slow continuous conduction. To all of this, time must be added for the impulse to be propagated across the neuromuscular junction and set up a compound muscle action potential (CMAP). Conduction along the muscle fibres can be disregarded since, once generated, the compound muscle action potential appears instantaneously by volume conduction.

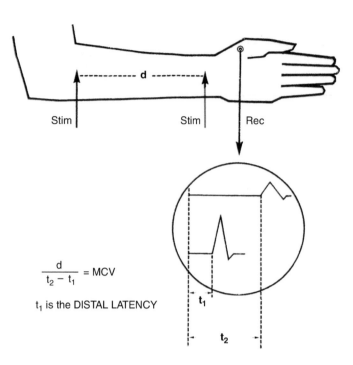

Diagram 12.2 Measurement of distal latency and motor conduction velocity. (Image included with permission from the Sheffield Teaching Hospitals NHS Foundation Trust.)

$$\frac{d}{t_2 - t_1} = MCV$$

t_1 is the DISTAL LATENCY

If we want to measure conduction velocity in motor nerves, we get round this problem by stimulating the nerve at two sites. The time interval between the stimulus and the appearance of the muscle response is called the latency. As with sensory studies, the stimulus produces an instantaneous artefact. Volume conduction analysis tells us that in the case of a CMAP recorded by surface electrodes, there will no initial positive wave, only a negative onset if the active electrode is located over the end-plate zone. An initial positive onset could indicate that the CMAP is arising from another muscle. Careful positioning is therefore called for. If necessary, a needle recording electrode should be used instead of surface electrodes to ensure the correct origin of the response, as discussed in Chapter 7, 'Some Technical Matters; Electrodes'.

In Diagram 12.2 the time interval between stimulation at the proximal site and the onset of the CMAP is called the proximal latency, t_2. Similarly, the time interval between the stimulus at the distal site and the CMAP onset is the distal latency, t_1. The difference between t_2 and t_1 gives us the conduction time over the distance, d, between the two stimulus sites, from which the motor conduction velocity (MCV) can be calculated.

The distal latency can be adjusted for distance but generally it is just used unmodified. It is often a very valuable measurement most notably in the diagnosis of carpal tunnel syndrome.

A couple of caveats need to be mentioned here. First, because a needle recording electrode will only pick up activity from closely adjacent tissue, it is possible that the motor nerve fibres supplying it may not be the largest diameter ones and so the measured MCV may not be the maximal MCV of the nerve. Second, the amplitude of the evoked response, the compound muscle action potential (CMAP), will be hugely dependent on the type and position of the recording electrode. Small changes in position of a needle recording electrode can produce large changes in the amplitude of the CMAP. Similarly, the locations of surface recording electrodes, both the active and the indifferent ones, have a significant though somewhat lesser influence on the amplitude of the recorded potential.

For these reasons, the amplitude of the CMAP, usually measured baseline to negative peak, is much less helpful in motor nerve conduction studies than is the amplitude of a SNAP in sensory studies. However, because the CMAPs are so much larger than SNAPs, abnormalities in their form may be more readily seen.

Amplitude and Form: The Effect of Conduction Distance

So far, we have been considering peripheral nerves as if they behaved in a fairly uniform manner. But as described in Chapter 3, 'Peripheral Nerve Types; Peripheral Nerve Classification', we have seen that they contain fibres of different diameters. And we have also seen in Chapter 4, 'Peripheral Nerve Function', that sodium ions, crucial to nerve conduction, flow along the interior of the nerve. So, the larger the diameter of the nerve, the less the internal resistance to this flow and thus the greater the conduction velocity. The effect on the amplitude and form of the recorded action potentials caused by conduction in fibres of different diameters is shown in Diagram 12.3.

Let us first consider what happens in a sensory or mixed nerve study. Supramaximal stimulation of the nerve at **A** is analogous to the firing of a starting pistol. Nerve action potentials are set up in all the myelinated nerves. They then travel towards the recording electrode at different velocities. If the distance travelled is short, as at **B**, there will be

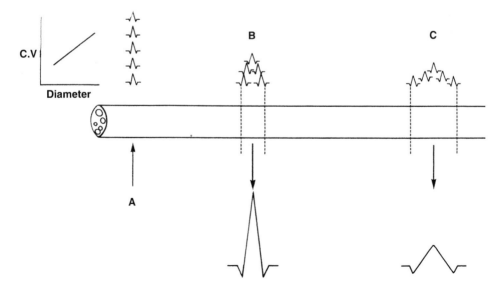

Diagram 12.3 The effect of different conduction velocities on the amplitude of the recorded nerve action potential. (Image included with permission from the Sheffield Teaching Hospitals NHS Foundation Trust.)

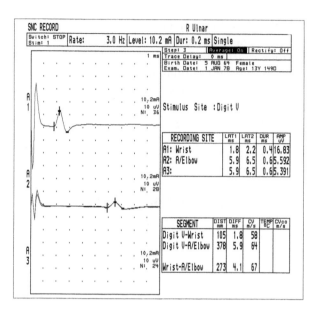

Figure 12.1 A normal ulnar nerve sensory conduction study. (Image included with permission from the Sheffield Teaching Hospitals NHS Foundation Trust.)

relatively little difference between the arrival times of the nerve action potentials from the fastest and the slowest conducting fibres. Their near-synchronous summation at the recording electrode will produce a SNAP (or MNAP) resembling a Gothic spire. If, however, the recording distance is considerable, as at C, there will be a correspondingly bigger difference between the arrival times of the nerve action potentials from the fastest and the slowest conducting fibres. This causes a spreading out or temporal dispersion of the recorded nerve action potentials so that the Gothic spire becomes more like a Norman arch. If the conduction distance is sufficiently long, the SNAP (or MNAP) may be unrecordable even in normal subjects.

An example of a normal ulnar nerve sensory conduction study is shown in Figure 12.1. In this and similar conduction studies the sweep speed is given at the top right-hand corner of the left pane. In relation to each tracing, the stimulus strength is shown in milliamps (mA) above the amplifier gain given in microVolts (μV) or milliVolts (mV). Below these, in sensory studies, the number of recordings averaged (*N*) is stated. To the right, the stimulus site is indicated in sensory studies. In motor studies the name of the muscle and the type of recording electrode used – surface electrodes (SE) or a concentric needle electrode (CNE) – are specified. The tabulated data are self-explanatory.

Because of this effect of conduction distance on amplitude, and because sensory nerve action potentials do not embody the natural advantages of the amplification factor seen in compound muscle action potentials, we need to use signal averagers in most cases of sensory and in some mixed nerve studies in order to record and clearly visualise the form of the recorded potential.

In normal subjects, the CMAPs are in the region of a thousand times larger than the SNAPs or MNAPs and so signal averagers are not required to observe that a similar effect is also happening here. It is also much less marked in motor studies

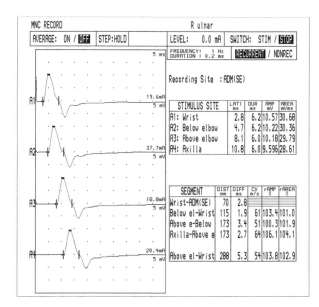

Figure 12.2 A normal ulnar nerve motor conduction study. (Image included with permission from the Sheffield Teaching Hospitals NHS Foundation Trust.)

because the range of conduction velocities in motor nerve fibres is less than the range in the sensory ones.

This effect in a normal ulnar motor nerve conduction study is shown in Figure 12.2 (please note the reduced gain compared with the sensory study). As the stimulus site is moved proximally, the amplitude of the CMAP diminishes slightly. The slight, apparent, relative slowing registered across the elbow is likely to be due to an underestimate of the conduction distance which has been measured with the elbow extended rather than flexed. The value recorded here is well within the normal range for the technique.

You will notice that the stimulus strength remains unaltered during the sensory study but is different at the different stimulus sites in the motor one. Once a supramaximal stimulus has been reached when stimulating a sensory nerve, it remains supramaximal irrespective of the location of the recording electrodes. However, in a motor study, a supramaximal stimulus must be delivered at more than one site. Because the impedance at each will vary, the examiner must be prepared to increase the stimulus strength until the amplitude of the CMAP ceases to grow.

Errors Caused by Submaximal Stimulation

If the stimulus strength is not supramaximal, false diagnostic inferences may be drawn from the results. For example, in the examination shown in Figure 12.3, the stimulus at the wrist in the lowest trace (A3) is clearly submaximal as evidenced by the small CMAP. The stimulus strength was 7.1 mA. That the largest diameter fibres have not been stimulated is shown by the long distal latency of 4.9 ms compared to the 3.4 ms obtained when the nerve was stimulated supramaximally at the same location, trace (A1). As a result, the apparent

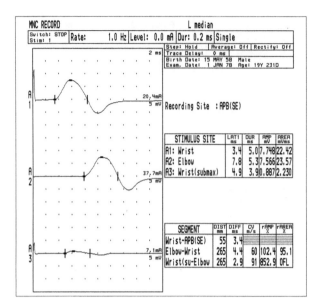

Figure 12.3 Submaximal stimulation causing false measurement of motor conduction velocity. (Image included with permission from the Sheffield Teaching Hospitals NHS Foundation Trust.)

conduction time between wrist and elbow is falsely short, 2.9 ms rather than the correct value of 4.4 ms, leading in turn to a falsely high conduction velocity of 91 m/s and not the correct value of 60 m/s.

Similarly, it can be shown that if the proximal stimulus is submaximal, the calculated conduction velocity will be falsely low.

Chapter 13

Nerve Conduction Studies: Degeneration

As we have seen in Chapter 2, 'Basic Anatomy and a Little Physiology', the peripheral nerve is part of the nerve cell body, just an extravagantly extruded extension of it. As such, it relies on metabolic processes taking place in the cell body for its healthy survival. When these begin to fail as a result of systemic or toxic disease, these most dependent parts of the cell will be the first to suffer. The process is called axonal degeneration.

This explains why, in degenerating peripheral neuropathies, we find the earliest changes in the extremities of the nerves. This is also why the longest nerves are the first to feel the effect. Clinically, symptoms affect the feet before the hands. With progressive disease, the pathology extends centripetally. This gives rise to the notion of 'dying-back' neuropathy. Because the Schwann cells which myelinate the axon are physically supported by it, degeneration results in loss of both components.

The same pathological changes may occur distal to the lesion after trauma. Diagram 13.1 shows distal degeneration in three myelinated nerve fibres from the largest diameter down to the smallest together with the position of the stimulating and recording electrodes applied to them. The recorded individual nerve action potentials and the

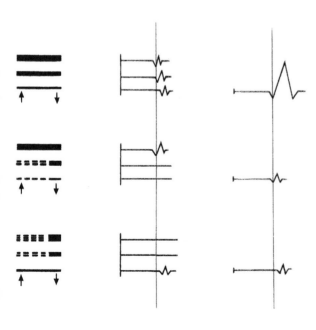

Diagram 13.1 The effect of degeneration in different diameter fibres on nerve conduction. (Image included with permission from the Sheffield Teaching Hospitals NHS Foundation Trust.)

algebraic summation of these appear to the right. Conditions are normal in the first case. In the second, there is degeneration (represented by discontinuous lines) sparing the largest diameter fibres, and in the last the pathology is involving all but the smallest diameter fibres.

Individual nerve fibres which are within the affected nerve but uninvolved by the pathology continue to conduct normally. The maximal conduction velocity will depend on the diameter of the largest survivors. It is possible, then, that in the early stages this velocity will be normal. As the largest diameter fibres are lost, so there will be corresponding slowing.

A way of visualising this is to consider a 'sinking' normal distribution curve. A normal distribution curve representing the range of conduction velocities is shown at **a** in Diagram 13.2. If nerves are lost in a fairly uniform manner the curve could be considered to sink, as at **b**, leading to a loss of the larger-diameter fibres and therefore a reduction in maximal conduction velocity.

Ingenious but clinically imperfect techniques have been devised to assess the range of normal conduction velocities in peripheral nerves. As a general rule of thumb, if the only remaining fibres are of the smallest diameter there will be a reduction in maximal conduction velocity of about 30%. Certainly, reductions significantly in excess of this indicate demyelination.

As we shall see, measurement of conduction velocity can be crucial in localising demyelinating lesions. But if the pathology is due to degeneration, studies of nerve conduction velocity are of limited value in this respect.

Diagram 13.3 compares the effects of lesions proximal or distal to the dorsal root ganglion. When the lesion is proximal to the bipolar dorsal root ganglion, as in cervical or lumber radiculopathy, the degenerating fibres (depicted as a discontinuous line) involve only those belonging to the central projections from the dorsal root ganglion and so the amplitude of the SNAP will be normal. But if degeneration affects the nerve distal to the dorsal root ganglion there will be loss of fibres leading to a corresponding reduction in the amplitude of the SNAP.

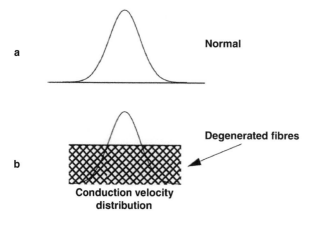

Diagram 13.2 Slowed conduction velocity due to loss of fibres. The effect on the normal distribution curve of fibre diameters (a) of uniform loss of fibres due to degeneration (b). (Illustration by author.)

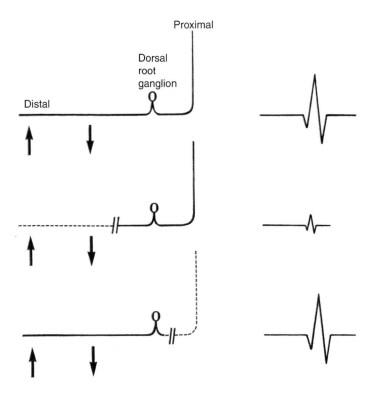

Diagram 13.3 Pathology proximal to the dorsal root does not affect the amplitude of the sensory nerve action potential. (Image included with permission from the Sheffield Teaching Hospitals NHS Foundation Trust.)

Beyond this, nerve conduction studies have little to offer in localising the watershed between the normal nerve and its degenerated distal component. In lesions following trauma this is hardly necessary. Diagram 13.4 illustrates this limitation.

As long as either the stimulating or recording electrodes are located over an affected section of the nerve, the reduced number of nerve fibres stimulated or recorded from will be reflected in a reduction in the amplitude of the SNAP or MNAP.

The poor localising capabilities of nerve conduction studies in degenerating neuropathy are offset, fortunately, by the availability of EMG. We have seen how this can diagnose degeneration by the demonstration of a reduced recruitment pattern and the presence of denervation potentials, such as fibrillation and positive sharp waves. Furthermore, the recording of abnormally long duration motor unit potentials indicate motor nerve regeneration and thus prior degeneration.

Examining different muscles with a view to identifying which peripheral nerve or myotome is affected requires the examiner to have a competent grasp of neuroanatomy as well as clinical neurology.

Despite this litany of limitations, nerve conduction studies in peripheral nerve degeneration are a very valuable clinical asset. The reduction in the number of functioning nerve fibres will lead to a corresponding reduction in the amplitude of the SNAP or MNAP. In other words, providing we are confident that a reduced potential is not due to conduction block, as discussed in Chapter 14 'Nerve Conduction Studies: Demyelination; Conduction Block', it provides a reliable and objective guide to the degree of degeneration present. In

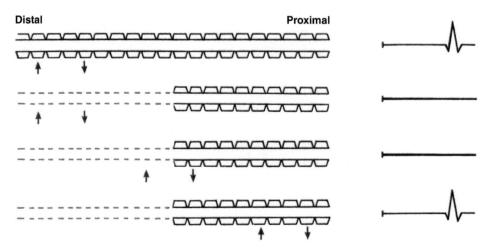

Distal   **Proximal**

Diagram 13.4 The limited capacity of nerve conduction studies to localise degeneration. (Image included with permission from the Sheffield Teaching Hospitals NHS Foundation Trust.)

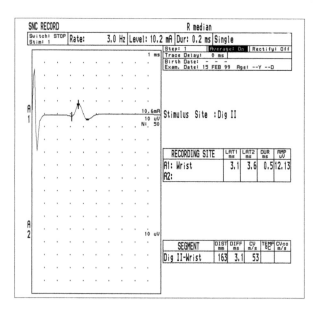

Figure 13.1 A normal median sensory nerve action potential. (Image included with permission from the Sheffield Teaching Hospitals NHS Foundation Trust.)

this way, the degree of pathology can be measured and, in theory at least, monitored. The amplitude of the CMAP is a less reliable indicator, being heavily dependent on technical factors as we have already seen in Chapter 12, 'Nerve Conduction Studies: Normal; Normal Motor Conduction Studies'. In Figure 13.1, we see an example of a normal SNAP recorded from a median nerve.

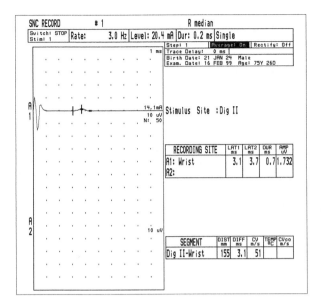

SNC RECORD	# 1		R median	
Switch: STOP Stim: 1	Rate:	3.0 Hz	Level: 20.4 mA	Dur: 0.2 ms	Single

	Step: 1	Average: On	Rectify: Off
	Trace Delay: 0 ms
	Birth Date: 21 JAN 24 Male
	Exam. Date: 16 FEB 99 Age: 75Y 26D

14, 1mA
10 uV
N:, 50

Stimulus Site :Dig II

RECORDING SITE	LAT1 ms	LAT2 ms	DUR ms	AMP uV
A1: Wrist	3.1	3.7	0.7	1.732
A2:				

SEGMENT	DIST mm	DIFF ms	CV m/s	TEMP ºC	CVco m/s
Dig II-Wrist	155	3.1	51		

Figure 13.2 A median sensory nerve action potential of reduced amplitude. (Image included with permission from the Sheffield Teaching Hospitals NHS Foundation Trust.)

Figure 13.2 shows a SNAP, also recorded from a median nerve, of considerably reduced amplitude but associated with a normal maximal sensory conduction velocity The finding implies severe degeneration which is probably sparing the larger diameter fibres.

Nerve Conduction Studies: Demyelination

14

Because myelin forms a discontinuous sheath around the nerve, demyelination may affect many segments on one nerve or many segments on many nerves. The first of these is characteristic of entrapment neuropathies; the second, of generalised demyelinating peripheral neuropathies.

Demyelination causes slowed conduction. This may be localised, as typified in entrapment neuropathies, or widespread as in demyelinating peripheral neuropathies. If the degree of demyelination is severe, conduction will fail altogether. This is because loss of myelin leads to an increase in the number of voltage-gated sodium channels exposed and hence a correspondingly reduced concentration, and thus effectiveness, of the finite number of depolarising sodium ions.

Demyelination may affect individual peripheral nerve fibres of different diameters differently. Diagram 14.1 is offered as a rather oversimplified aid to understanding how these differences produce different electrophysiological effects.

Each section in the diagram shows three myelinated nerve fibres from the largest diameter down to the smallest, together with the position of the stimulating and recording electrodes applied to them. The recorded potentials, both the individual nerve action potentials and the algebraic summation of them, appear to the right.

Normal conditions are seen in the first example. Next, we see demyelination, as represented by the thin segment, affecting all nerves equally. Maximal conduction velocity will be slowed but the potential will be normal in amplitude and form. In the third example, demyelination is affecting the smaller diameter fibres but sparing the largest ones. Again, maximal conduction velocity will be normal but the potential will be desynchronised and therefore also correspondingly reduced in amplitude. In the final example, there is severe demyelination sufficient to cause conduction block, as represented by the gap, in all but the largest diameter fibres. This results in a reduction in the amplitude of the potential but the maximal conduction velocity will be normal.

Of course, these basic categories of abnormality – slowing of maximal conduction velocity, desynchronisation and conduction block – frequently co-exist in different combinations to different degrees.

We will now look at examples of how these pathologies may be inferred from the electrophysiological findings in patients with nerve entrapment – a bountiful hunting ground for the clinical neurophysiologist.

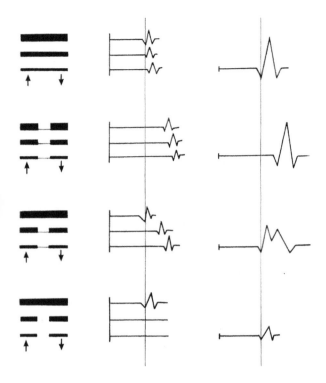

Diagram 14.1 The effect of demyelination in different diameter fibres on nerve conduction. (Image included with permission from the Sheffield Teaching Hospitals NHS Foundation Trust.)

Slowed Conduction in the Largest Diameter Fibres

First, in Figure 14.1, we see an example of normal maximal sensory conduction velocity in the median nerve between dig II and wrist.

By contrast, Figure 14.2 shows an example of slowed maximal sensory conduction velocity in a patient with carpal tunnel syndrome.

You can see that, in addition to slowing of maximal sensory conduction velocity, the amplitude of the SNAP is reduced. This could be due to slowing or conduction block in smaller diameter fibres and/or degeneration in them. If the latter is occurring, there will probably also be motor nerve degeneration which can be diagnosed by electromyography.

We have seen that, in motor studies, we measure conduction velocity and distal latency. A distal lesion, such as carpal tunnel syndrome, will show normal conduction between elbow and wrist but slowing between wrist and muscle. Figure 14.3 shows a normal median nerve motor study to abductor pollicis brevis, which is the usually chosen recording site as it is the only intrinsic muscle of the hand innervated exclusively by the median nerve:

Figure 14.4 is taken from an examination of a patient with carpal tunnel syndrome showing normal conduction between elbow and wrist but a prolonged distal latency.

Slowed Conduction in Smaller Diameter Fibres

Because of the normally small ulnar nerve SNAP recorded at above-elbow, motor studies tend to be more useful in the diagnosis of local entrapment of this nerve at the elbow. Nevertheless, this is not always the case and in the sensory study shown in Figure 14.5 there

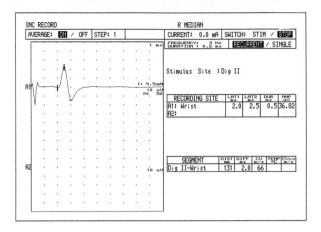

Figure 14.1 A normal median nerve sensory study. (Image included with permission from the Sheffield Teaching Hospitals NHS Foundation Trust.)

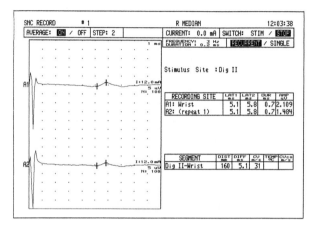

Figure 14.2 Slowed sensory conduction in a median nerve. (Image included with permission from the Sheffield Teaching Hospitals NHS Foundation Trust.)

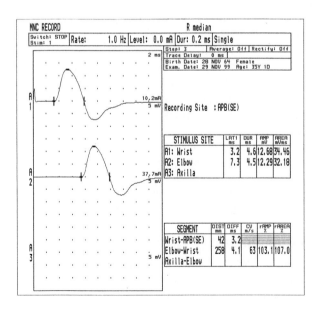

Figure 14.3 A normal median nerve motor study. (Image included with permission from the Sheffield Teaching Hospitals NHS Foundation Trust.)

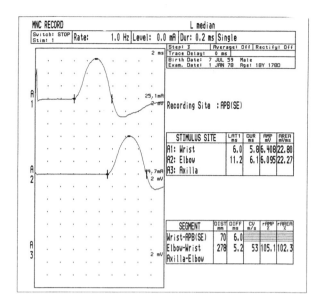

Figure 14.4 A median nerve motor study showing a prolonged distal latency to abductor pollicis brevis. (Image included with permission from the Sheffield Teaching Hospitals NHS Foundation Trust.)

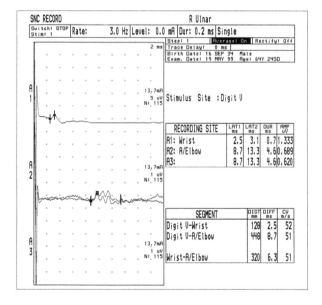

Figure 14.5 An ulnar nerve sensory study showing desynchronisation of the sensory nerve action potential recorded above the elbow. (Image included with permission from the Sheffield Teaching Hospitals NHS Foundation Trust.)

is normal conduction velocity in large-diameter fibres across the elbow but slowed conduction in smaller diameter fibres causing desynchronisation of the SNAP (please note the increased gain in the above-elbow study).

The considerably reduced amplitude of the SNAP recorded at the wrist in the context of normal conduction velocity over this segment is likely to be due to co-existent degeneration in many of the other fibres.

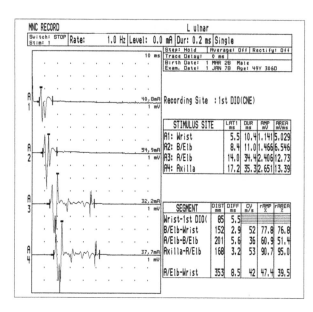

Figure 14.6 An ulnar nerve motor study showing slowed conduction across the elbow and desynchronisation of the compound muscle action potential when the nerve is stimulated proximal to the elbow. (Image included with permission from the Sheffield Teaching Hospitals NHS Foundation Trust.)

In Figure 14.6, we see an example of slowed maximal motor conduction velocity across the elbow in the ulnar nerve, indicating local entrapment. Also, when stimulating at above-elbow or axilla, there is a markedly desynchronised CMAP. The changes imply that slowing is present in the largest diameter fibres and even more so in the smaller ones.

Conduction Block

In Figure 14.7, we see an example of severe slowing of maximal motor conduction velocity across the elbow in the ulnar nerve and pronounced changes in the amplitude of the CMAPs recorded during stimulation at above-elbow and axilla.

Because the amplitudes of the CMAPs recorded during more distal stimulation are normal, implying normal numbers of conducting fibres between the stimulating and recording electrodes, the decrement seen during stimulation at more proximal sites indicates that there is conduction block at the elbow and its degree. A submaximal stimulus will generate a CMAP of reduced amplitude and so it is important to ensure that the stimulation is supramaximal.

Localisation of the Lesion

When these features – slowing, desynchronisation and/or conduction block – are encountered, we can be confident that the lesion lies somewhere between the stimulating and recording electrodes. Diagram 14.2 illustrates the principle.

If the degree of slowing is mild, its detection may be obscured by normal conduction over segments adjacent to the demyelinated region. This diluting effect, which poses a common diagnostic difficulty in the identification of entrapment neuropathies, is clearly proportional to the length of normal nerve between the electrodes. Therefore, we try to keep the inter-electrode distance as short as possible over the area of interest. For example, in

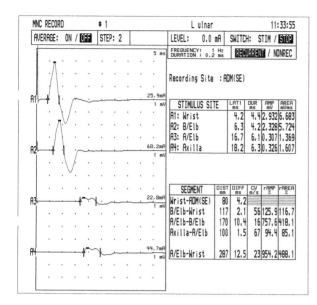

MNC RECORD   # 1   L ulnar   11:33:55

AVERAGE: ON / OFF   STEP: 2   LEVEL: 0.0 mA   SWITCH: STIM / STOP
                                        5 ms   FREQUENCY: 1 Hz   RECURRENT / NONREC
                                               DURATION : 0.2 ms

Recording Site : ADM(SE)

STIMULUS SITE	LAT1 ms	DUR ms	AMP mV	AREA mVms
A1: Wrist	4.2	4.4	2.932	6.683
A2: B/Elb	6.3	4.2	2.328	5.724
A3: A/Elb	16.7	6.1	0.307	1.369
A4: Axilla	18.2	6.3	0.326	1.607

SEGMENT	DIST mm	DIFF ms	CV m/s	rAMP %	rAREA %
Wrist-ADM(SE)	80	4.2			
B/Elb-Wrist	117	2.1	56	125.9	116.7
A/Elb-B/Elb	170	10.4	16	757.6	418.1
Axilla-A/Elb	100	1.5	67	94.4	85.1
A/Elb-Wrist	287	12.5	23	954.2	488.1

A1   25.9mA 1 mV
A2   68.2mA 1 mV
A3   22.8mA 1 mV
A4   44.7mA 1 mV

Figure 14.7 An ulnar nerve motor study showing marked slowing and conduction block across the elbow. (Image included with permission from the Sheffield Teaching Hospitals NHS Foundation Trust.)

Distal   Proximal

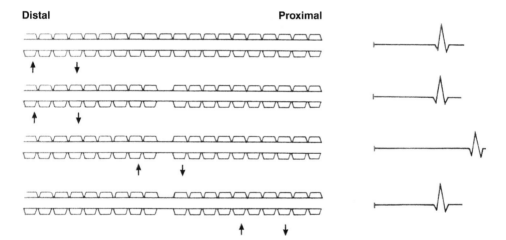

Diagram 14.2 How nerve conduction studies localise demyelination. (Image included with permission from the Sheffield Teaching Hospitals NHS Foundation Trust.)

ulnar nerve studies, we stimulate motor nerves at above and below the elbow, and, in the case of the peroneal nerve, at the popliteal fossa and head of the fibula.

The value of this strategy can be shown in the following examples during investigation of possible carpal tunnel syndrome. Digit III is stimulated and SNAPs recorded over the palm and the wrist. Careful attention to technique is called for as stimulus artefact can be troublesome at the recording from the palm. Selecting the longest digital nerve helps to minimise this. This technique often demonstrates slowing between palm and wrist in the

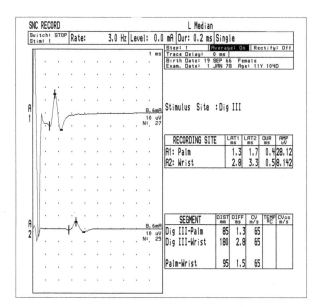

Figure 14.8 A normal median nerve sensory study, recording at the palm and the wrist. (Image included with permission from the Sheffield Teaching Hospitals NHS Foundation Trust.)

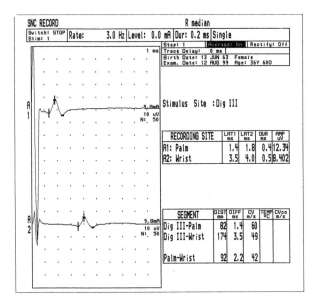

Figure 14.9 A median nerve sensory study showing slowed conduction between palm and wrist. (Image included with permission from the Sheffield Teaching Hospitals NHS Foundation Trust.)

context of normal conduction between digit and palm, and therefore the presence of a lesion when all other measurements are normal.

Figure 14.8 shows a normal examination.

And in Figure 14.9 we see a recording from a patient with a mild carpal tunnel syndrome.

The conduction velocity between digit III and wrist is no more than borderline slow, but it is clearly reduced between palm and wrist compared against the normal conduction velocity between digit and palm.

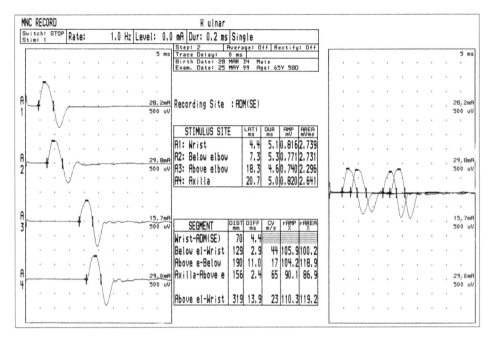

Figure 14.10 An ulnar nerve motor study from a patient with entrapment of the nerve at the elbow. (Image included with permission from the Sheffield Teaching Hospitals NHS Foundation Trust.)

Similarly, in the motor study of the ulnar nerve shown in Figure 14.10, there is clear and marked slowing across the elbow.

The small amplitudes of the CMAPs and the borderline slowing between below-elbow and wrist indicate that pathology in some of the fibres has progressed to degeneration.

Superimposition of the traces on the right emphasises the degree and location of the slowed conduction.

Chapter 15

Degree of Pathology

In Chapter 14, 'Nerve Conduction Studies: Demyelination', we have seen that demyelination causes slowed conduction in the affected nerve fibre. This is proportional to the degree of pathology. More severe pathology leads to conduction block.

We have also talked about myelin acting as an insulator around the nerve fibre in Chapter 4, 'Peripheral Nerve Function'. If insulation is stripped from an electrical cable, conduction will continue. But in a nerve, it will not. This is because nerve impulse propagation requires a minimum density of sodium ions to depolarise the membrane. Severe loss of myelin segments will dilute the concentration of sodium ions over the affected region.

A severely demyelinated nerve fibre is also unstable. The portion of nerve distal to a focal lesion may undergo axonal degeneration. These effects, particularly the reduction in the amplitude of SNAPs and the findings of denervation and/or regeneration on electromyography, are valuable in assessing the degree of pathology.

By way of illustration, let us consider the case of ulnar entrapment at the elbow. As the degree of entrapment increases, so does the degree of local demyelination. Slowing in affected fibres increases and ultimately there is conduction block. However, providing the pathology remains demyelinating in character and therefore local, normal conditions will be found distally. But as the degree of demyelination increases, the nerve fibre undergoes degeneration distal to the lesion. This is shown in Diagram 15.1.

In the first example, we assume that there is severe demyelination and maybe even conduction block at the elbow. The lesion is represented by the thin segment. But the pathology is still not sufficiently severe to cause nerve fibres to degenerate. So a normal amplitude SNAP will be recorded at the wrist during stimulation of digit V. In the second and third cases the lesion has become sufficiently severe to lead to progressively more axonal degeneration, as represented by the discontinuous line, distal to the lesion. The SNAP recorded at the wrist will be reduced in amplitude in proportion to the degree of degeneration.

In assessing the degree of degeneration, whether secondary to demyelination as shown or arising de novo, we must now acknowledge some shortcomings. Because the distribution of SNAP amplitudes in normal subjects is positively skewed, significant fibre loss may sometimes be reliably inferred only when fairly extreme.

Scrutiny of CMAP amplitudes suffer similar drawbacks. More crucially, their considerable dependence on the position of the active and indifferent recording electrodes severely constrains their contribution to the assessment of the degree of pathology.

Fibrillation and positive sharp wave activity would indicate that degeneration has occurred and, if profuse, imply severe degeneration. As has already been discussed in

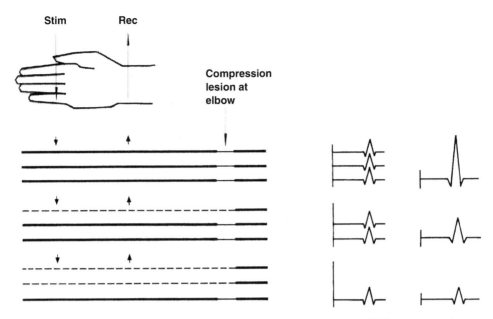

Diagram 15.1 A distal ulnar sensory study showing the effects of proximal lesions of different degrees. (Image included with permission from the Sheffield Teaching Hospitals NHS Foundation Trust.)

Chapter 10, 'Electromyography (EMG)', there is no satisfactory method of quantifying the recruitment pattern. Nevertheless, when this is clearly reduced, it tends to correlate fairly well with the degree of axonal degeneration. If the lesion is chronic, the finding of long-duration MUPs implying regeneration is a valuable indicator that degeneration has occurred but a poor guide to its degree.

The identification of the prevailing pathology is important because recovery from demyelination is relatively rapid depending upon local Schwann cells wrapping themselves around surviving axons but recovery from degeneration is a very different matter. The nerve must regrow and be remyelinated. The rate of recovery is commonly said to be 1 mm per day but regrowth may not start straight away and the time required to make distal connections, particularly to muscles, must also be factored into the calculation.

Monitoring

For an objective and quantitative technique, the limited capability of electrophysiological methods to monitor change is perhaps surprising but definitely disappointing. However, after a severe lesion, EMG findings will sometimes indicate that recovery is occurring long before it is clinically evident.

Degenerated nerve fibres have a great propensity for recovery even though it is by the slow process of regeneration. The newly formed nerve fibres are extremely thin at first and the remyelinated segments are also shorter than normal. Conduction along them is slow, often spectacularly so. As more nerve fibres regenerate, so there are more individual nerve action potentials contributing to the SNAP, MNAP or CMAP amplitudes.

However, recovery is generally much more easily recognised in motor than sensory fibres by using EMG rather than NCS, capitalising on the amplification properties of the motor unit potential. The very small MUPs formed by a few regenerating nerve sprouts after severe degeneration are not only reduced in amplitude but are also usually polyphasic in form. They are called nascent potentials. Increased jitter, which is also commonly seen, indicates that their end-plates are immature. Jitter is a measure of the stability of neuro-muscular transmission and will be discussed in detail in Chapter 16, 'Tests of Neuromuscular Transmission'.

These small polyphasic potentials, shown in a free-running trace in Figure 15.1, were recorded from a patient who had sustained a severe brachial plexus injury.

Using trigger and delay facilities, increasing the gain of the amplifier, and adjusting its filter settings allow us to inspect the components of one of these potentials, as shown in Figure 15.2.

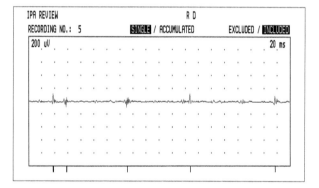

Figure 15.1 Nascent motor unit potentials indicating motor nerve regeneration. (Image included with permission from the Sheffield Teaching Hospitals NHS Foundation Trust.)

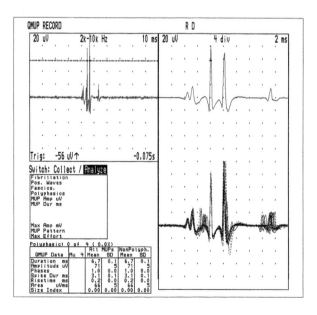

Figure 15.2 A nascent motor unit potential showing instability of its components. (Image included with permission from the Sheffield Teaching Hospitals NHS Foundation Trust.)

If we look at the superimposed recordings from repetitive firings of the motor unit, seen at the bottom of the right-hand panel, the second largest spike which has been used to trigger the trace remains stable. All other spike components of this MUP show varying degrees of blurring corresponding the variability of neuromuscular transmission. In some cases the baseline is seen through an outline of faint, fuzzy spikes. This indicates intermittent failure of neuromuscular transmission across the end-plate which is called blocking. But good clinical skills remain the cornerstone of monitoring recovery.

Chapter 16

Tests of Neuromuscular Transmission

Some details of the structure and function of the neuromuscular junction have been described earlier in Chapter 5, 'The Neuromuscular Junction'.

Acetylcholine (ACh) molecules are packaged in units called quanta within vesicles inside the nerve terminal. There is a pool of vesicles, the primary pool, very close to the synaptic membrane, ready to release their contents by the process of exocytosis. Close by is a secondary pool which can be mobilised to replenish the primary pool. This may take 1 or 2 seconds. Additional sources of ACh backing up these two are to be found in the axon and cell body.

Nerve impulses depolarising the terminal increase the inflow of calcium (Ca) through voltage-gated channels. The inflow is minimal at low firing rates but substantial at high firing rates. Calcium within the nerve terminal promotes the exocytosis of the vesicles and thus the release of ACh molecules into the synaptic cleft. Here they combine with the ACh receptors on the muscle membrane which open the sodium channels leading to depolarisation.

Repetitive Nerve Stimulation (RNS)

We are now in a position to understand what happens when a motor nerve is stimulated at low or high repetition rates whilst recording a compound muscle action potential (CMAP) from the muscle it supplies.

Myasthenia Gravis

In myasthenia gravis, MG, the pathology is post-synaptic. Antibodies against ACh receptors on the muscle fibres block or destroy them. Despite the loss of functioning ACh receptors, the safety factor usually ensures that a single stimulus to the motor nerve will discharge sufficient ACh to produce end-plate potentials (EPPs) in enough muscle fibres to summate to form a normal amplitude CMAP.

At slow rates of stimulation, less than 5 Hz, the initial CMAP will be of normal amplitude but after 1 or 2 seconds the amount of ACh being released from the primary store has diminished. The amount may now be insufficient to depolarise enough receptors in the abnormal end-plates in some muscle fibres. These will no longer contribute a muscle action potential to the CMAP, which will therefore show some decrement. The decrement is seldom much greater than the 10% required for diagnosis.

Figure 16.1 shows a study of normal neuromuscular transmission. A sequence of CMAPs recorded from abductor pollicis brevis following repeated stimulation of the median nerve at the wrist is shown. The repetition frequency of the stimulus can be seen

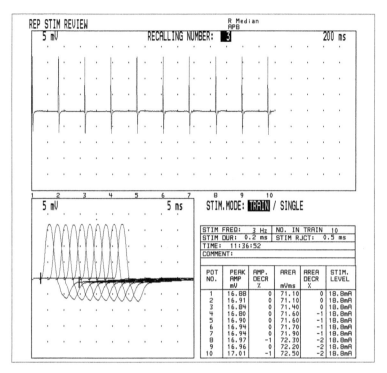

REP STIM REVIEW   R Median APB

5 mV   RECALLING NUMBER: 3   200 ms

5 mV   5 ms   STIM.MODE: TRAIN / SINGLE

STIM FREQ:	3 Hz	NO. IN TRAIN	10
STIM DUR:	0.2 ms	STIM RJCT:	0.5 ms
TIME:	11:36:52		
COMMENT:			

POT NO.	PEAK AMP mV	AMP. DECR %	AREA mVms	AREA DECR %	STIM. LEVEL
1	16.88	0	71.10	0	18.8mA
2	16.91	0	71.10	0	18.8mA
3	16.84	0	71.40	0	18.8mA
4	16.80	0	71.60	-1	18.8mA
5	16.90	0	71.60	-1	18.8mA
6	16.94	0	71.70	-1	18.8mA
7	16.94	0	71.90	-1	18.8mA
8	16.97	-1	72.30	-2	18.8mA
9	16.96	0	72.20	-2	18.8mA
10	17.01	-1	72.50	-2	18.8mA

Figure 16.1 Repetitive nerve stimulation in a normal subject. (Image included with permission from the Sheffield Teaching Hospitals NHS Foundation Trust.)

to be 3 Hz. The gains in each window are the same but the sweep speed is faster in the lower window and the potentials have been partially overlapped to aid the assessment of possible decrement.

In Figure 16.2 we see the result from a similar study in a patient with myasthenia gravis. There is the typical initial decrement which then stabilises, thought to be the result of mobilisation of ACh from the secondary pool.

At high rates of stimulation, the compensatory influence of Ca influx in increasing the release of ACh may result in a normal, non-decrementing response. But in more severe cases, the compensation is insufficient and a decrementing response will also be seen.

If no significant decrement is recorded, the test of post-exercise exhaustion may be tried. Intermittent RNS continues for several minutes after a prolonged period of maximal voluntary contraction. The voluntary effort may increase the stress of transmission across the neuromuscular junction and yield a positive result.

If there has been a decremental response to RNS, when the stimulation is repeated after a short period of maximal effort there may be some recovery in the size of the CMAP. This is known as post-exercise facilitation. It has been ascribed to an increased release of ACh as a result of Ca influx to the nerve following the intense voluntary effort.

Unfortunately, this technique and that of post-exercise exhaustion are, in the author's view, seldom helpful. Thus, if there has been a decremental response to RNS, further RNS testing is unlikely to add clinically useful information. If there has been no decrement, it is

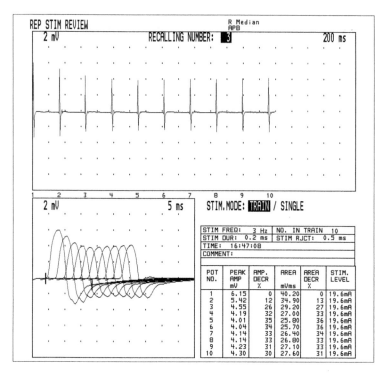

Figure 16.2 Repetitive nerve stimulation in a patient with myasthenia gravis showing initial decrement in the amplitude of the compound muscle action potential. (Image included with permission from the Sheffield Teaching Hospitals NHS Foundation Trust.)

usually more profitable to proceed to single-fibre electromyography (SFEMG) than to persist with more RNS studies.

Myasthenia gravis tends to affect proximal rather than distal limb muscles and facial muscles even more so. Although modified techniques have been devised to allow the application of RNS studies to these muscles, SFEMG remains the preferred option by many if peripheral testing is negative.

Myasthenic Syndrome (Lambert–Eaton Myasthenic Syndrome, LEMS)

In Lambert–Eaton myasthenic syndrome the pathology is pre-synaptic. Insufficient vesicles are released to depolarise all the end-plates of the muscle fibres innervated by the nerve, with the result that the CMAP may be reduced in amplitude.

At low rates of stimulation, which further reduce the output of ACh from the primary store of vesicles after about 1 to 2 seconds, there will be a decrementing response in what is often an abnormally small initial CMAP.

Figure 16.3 shows an example of typical findings in this condition. Initially, groups of ten stimuli were given at different rates, namely 1, 2, 3, 5, 10 and 1 Hz. The upper window shows the amplitudes of the recorded CMAPs, represented as solid columns, for the sequence of each group of stimuli. The lower window displays the potentials from one group at a faster sweep speed and partially overlapped.

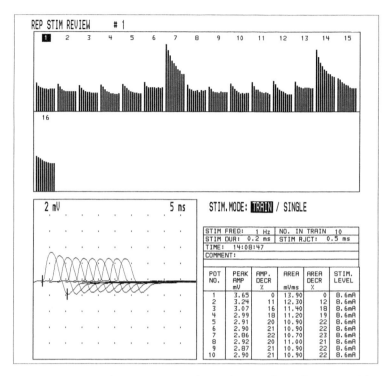

REP STIM REVIEW # 1

STIM.MODE: TRAIN / SINGLE

STIM FREQ:	1 Hz	NO. IN TRAIN	10
STIM DUR:	0.2 ms	STIM RJCT:	0.5 ms
TIME:	14:08:47		
COMMENT:			

POT NO.	PEAK AMP mV	AMP, DECR %	AREA mVms	AREA DECR %	STIM. LEVEL
1	3.65	0	13.90	0	8.6mA
2	3.24	11	12.30	12	8.6mA
3	3.07	16	11.40	18	8.6mA
4	2.99	18	11.20	19	8.6mA
5	2.91	20	10.90	22	8.6mA
6	2.90	21	10.90	22	8.6mA
7	2.86	22	10.70	23	8.6mA
8	2.92	20	11.00	21	8.6mA
9	2.87	21	10.90	22	8.6mA
10	2.90	21	10.90	22	8.6mA

Figure 16.3 Repetitive nerve stimulation in a patient with myasthenic syndrome showing initial decrement in the amplitude of the compound muscle action potential. (Study 1). (Image included with permission from the Sheffield Teaching Hospitals NHS Foundation Trust.)

The first study, during stimulation at 1 Hz, has been selected as shown by the white figure on the black background in the upper trace and by the STIM FREQ statement in the table. Data in the table also show that the peak amplitude of the first CMAP is rather small at 3.65 mV and that after a few seconds a decrement of over 20% occurs.

However, if high rates of stimulation of, say, 20 Hz or greater are administered, the influx of Ca promotes a dramatic increase in ACh release sufficient to depolarise the end-plates of many otherwise quiescent muscle fibres. These summate in an incrementing CMAP response of 100% or more.

Stimulation at these rates can be something of an eye-watering procedure for the patient. The desired effect on Ca behaviour can usually be just as easily and definitely more acceptably realised by asking the patient to make a short but maximal voluntary contraction of the muscle under examination before stimulating at a low repetition rate, as was the case here. So, after the first six trains of stimuli the patient was asked to make a sustained maximal voluntary contraction. This was immediately followed by a train of stimuli at 1 Hz. The result appears in Study 7 in Figure 16.4.

The increment is clearly well in excess of 100% (compare the peak amplitude of the first response in this train, 8.67 mV, with the first response of the initial train at 1 Hz as shown in Figure 16.3, namely 3.65 mV). The procedure was repeated to show reproducibility, a similar degree of increment being recorded in Study 14.

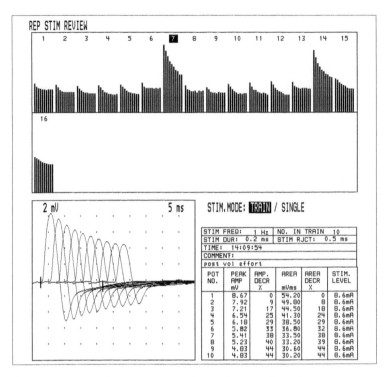

REP STIM REVIEW

STIM.MODE: **TRAIN** / SINGLE

STIM FREQ:	1 Hz	NO. IN TRAIN	10
STIM DUR:	0.2 ms	STIM RJCT:	0.5 ms
TIME:	14:09:54		
COMMENT:			
post vol effort			

POT NO.	PEAK AMP mV	AMP. DECR %	AREA mVms	AREA DECR %	STIM. LEVEL
1	8.67	0	54.20	0	8.6mA
2	7.92	9	49.80	8	8.6mA
3	7.21	17	44.50	18	8.6mA
4	6.54	25	41.30	24	8.6mA
5	6.18	29	38.50	29	8.6mA
6	5.82	33	36.80	32	8.6mA
7	5.41	38	33.50	38	8.6mA
8	5.23	40	33.20	39	8.6mA
9	4.83	44	30.60	44	8.6mA
10	4.83	44	30.20	44	8.6mA

2 mV   5 ms

Figure 16.4 Repetitive nerve stimulation in a patient with myasthenic syndrome showing over 100% increment in the amplitude of the compound muscle action potential after a short period of voluntary muscle contraction. (Study 7). That this effect is reproducible is shown in Study 14. (Image included with permission from the Sheffield Teaching Hospitals NHS Foundation Trust.)

A small incremental response, pseudofacilitation, may be seen in normal individuals. It has been attributed to a better degree of synchronisation of the individual muscle fibre action potentials. An example is shown in Figure 16.5.

Ten stimuli were given at different rates, in this case at 1, 2, 3, 5, 10, 1 and 1 Hz. As before, the upper trace shows the amplitudes of each CMAP represented as a solid column and the lower window shows the potentials from the selected study at a fast sweep speed and partially overlapped. In this case, Study 5 during stimulation at 10 Hz has been selected. It is clear that the slight squeezing of the form of the CMAPs has increased their amplitude.

Single-Fibre Electromyography (SFEMG)

There are two techniques of single-fibre electromyography (SFEMG), both designed to demonstrate variability in neuromuscular transmission time. This will be increased in pre- or post-junctional disorders of neuromuscular transmission because any late components will skew the normal distribution curve.

In stimulated SFEMG (sSFEMG), a motor nerve branch is stimulated to produce a muscle action potential in a single muscle fibre. In voluntary SFEMG (vSFEMG), MUPs from two fibres are recorded during voluntary contraction of the muscle. The advantages of

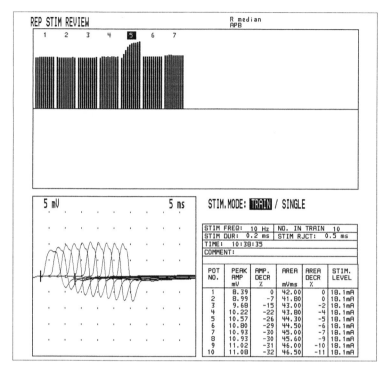

Figure 16.5 Repetitive nerve stimulation showing pseudofacilitation. (Image included with permission from the Sheffield Teaching Hospitals NHS Foundation Trust.)

sSFEMG are that it requires no voluntary effort from the patient and the effect of different stimulus frequencies can be investigated. The disadvantages are that selection of a satisfactory stimulus site may require the use of another needle electrode, and excessive stimulus strength may directly depolarise the muscle fibre, by-passing the neuromuscular junction. The advantage of vSFEMG is that it requires no initial set-up. The disadvantage is that it depends on sustained, steady and weak voluntary contraction of the muscle. Because the principles underlying both techniques are the same, and because the author has more experience of vSFEMG, this is the technique chosen to describe in more detail.

A needle electrode with a small recording area is manipulated so that it records from just two single muscle fibres. The delay at the neuromuscular junction between the arrival of the nerve action potential at the nerve terminal and the generation of a muscle action potential (MAP) will vary each time depending on how quickly vesicles are released and how long it takes for the ACh to bind to receptors and set up an action potential.

In Diagram 16.1, we imagine MAPs recorded from two normal single muscle fibres, A and B. The difference in their arrival times is determined principally by the distance of their end-plates from the recording electrode. But superimposed on this are subtle differences due to variability in the neuromuscular transmission time for each fibre. This variability can be considered to follow a normal distribution curve for each fibre.

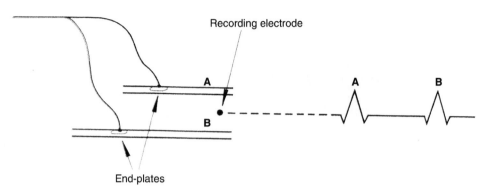

Diagram 16.1 The interpeak interval between the action potentials from two single muscle fibres is mainly due to the difference in distance of each end-plate from the recording electrode. (Image included with permission from the Sheffield Teaching Hospitals NHS Foundation Trust.)

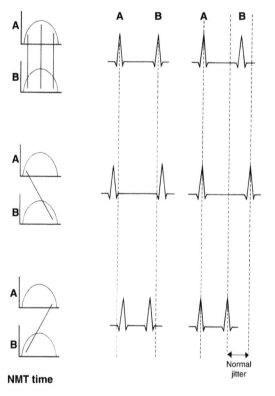

Diagram 16.2 Neuromuscular transmission at two normal end-plates gives a normal jitter value. NMT denotes neuromuscular transmission. (Image included with permission from the Sheffield Teaching Hospitals NHS Foundation Trust.)

In the first trace in Diagram 16.2, the potentials from both muscle fibres are generated at similar points on their respective normal neuromuscular transmission time (NMT time) distribution curves, which are depicted in a stylised form to aid explanation. Next, we consider that the potential at **A** arrives relatively early and at **B** relatively late. And then vice versa.

The different arrival times of the potentials are shown to the left. Superimposing the traces will be a meaningless blur but if we trigger the display using fibre **A** then the variability in neuromuscular transmission can be easily seen, as shown on the right. When the inter-potential interval is long, we can infer that either the action potential at **A** was early and/or the one at **B** was late. Likewise, a short interval denotes a late arrival at **A** and/or an early arrival at **B**. This variability is called jitter and can be quantified. We measure the interval between the two peaks for all pairs. We then note the absolute value of the difference between consecutive measurements. The average of these is descriptively called the mean consecutive difference, which is the jitter value.

Next, in Diagram 16.3, we see that the distribution curves are skewed showing an increase in the probability of delayed transmission.

Using the same explanations as before, it is clear that in the first two examples the inter-potential intervals are excessively long and excessively short, respectively, compared with the normal range, shown as the hatched area. In the third case, only muscle fibre **A** has generated an action potential to trigger the display. Neuromuscular transmission has failed in fibre **B**, a condition called blocking. A similar picture would of course be seen if, instead, the blocking had been in fibre **A**.

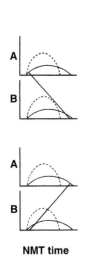

NMT time

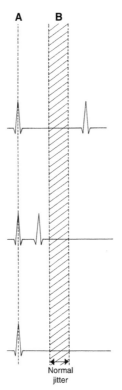

A   B

Diagram 16.3 Delayed neuromuscular transmission at two end-plates gives an increased jitter value. Transmission across only one end-plate causes blocking. NMT denotes neuromuscular transmission. (Image included with permission from the Sheffield Teaching Hospitals NHS Foundation Trust.)

Normal jitter

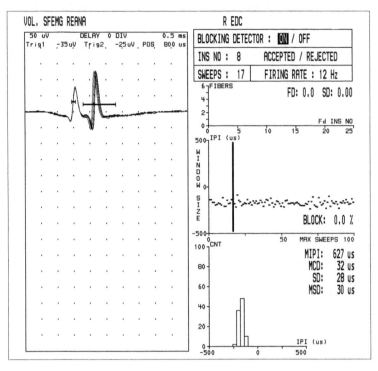

Figure 16.6 Single-fibre electromyography showing a normal jitter value. (Image included with permission from the Sheffield Teaching Hospitals NHS Foundation Trust.)

It has been assumed that neuromuscular transmission is abnormal at both end-plates. If only one were affected, jitter would be increased but less so.

An example of a normal clinical study is shown in Figure 16.6. The potentials from the repeated firing of two muscle fibres are seen. The amplifier gain is shown at the top left-hand corner of the left pane and the sweep speed at the top right-hand corner.

The first potential triggers the sweep and delay of the display. The arrival time of the second relative to it shows slight variability as evidenced by the slightly fuzzy outline. The computer calculates these values, the interpeak interval (the IPI), and plots them. From these values, the mean consecutive difference, MCD or jitter value, is derived. You can also see that if one muscle fibre is active, so is the other one. In other words there is no blocking. In myasthenia gravis. neuromuscular transmission may fail in one of the fibres, so-called conduction block. In such cases, only one potential will be recorded and this will trigger the display. The absence of the potential from the other, affected fibre in which neuromuscular transmission has failed can easily be inferred from the presence of an undisturbed baseline running through the second group of potentials.

Next, in Figure 16.7, we see a single-fibre study from a patient with myasthenia gravis. The arrival of the second potential relative to the first one is clearly more variable than in the normal case – and please note that the sweep speed has been reduced from 0.5 ms per division to 1 ms per division, otherwise the appearance would be even more striking. The

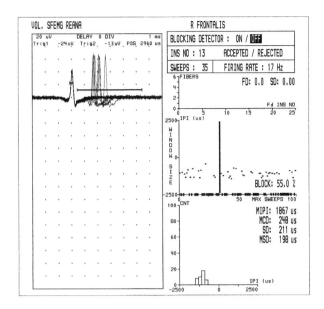

Figure 16.7 Single-fibre electromyography in a patient with myasthenia gravis showing markedly increased jitter and also blocking. (Image included with permission from the Sheffield Teaching Hospitals NHS Foundation Trust.)

MCD, the jitter value, is very much increased denoting abnormal neuromuscular transmission. A considerable degree of blocking is also evident.

It is probable that most, if not all, clinical neurophysiologists have congratulated themselves on coining the phrase 'all that jitters is not myasthenia'. If nothing else, it emphasis the veracity of the observation. For example, it is a particularly noteworthy finding in peripheral nerve regeneration where the end-plates are immature with consequent insecurity of neuromuscular transmission.

17 Other Techniques: F-waves and H-reflexes

F-wave Studies

If we stimulate a motor nerve supra-maximally, for example, the median nerve at the wrist, the wave of depolarisation travels orthodromically to the muscle to produce a compound muscle action potential. It also travels antidromically. When it reaches the anterior horn cell, what happens next depends on the excitatory state of the neuron. If it is close to firing, this antidromic input may be just enough to depolarise the cell and produce an action potential. The majority of cells within the motor neuron pool from which a peripheral nerve arises will be some way from firing threshold but a few may be sufficiently close to be susceptible.

The result is a late and small CMAP called the F-wave. Late because of the distance travelled in this round trip, and small because, at best, only one or a few anterior horn cells will be close to firing. If the stimulus is repeated, there may be no F-wave response because all anterior horn cells are in a relatively inexcitable state, or there may be an F-wave response with a different latency. This, in turn, may be due to a difference in the time taken to depolarise the anterior horn cell and/or conduction in a different diameter fibre with a different conduction velocity.

What is recorded is the normal CMAP, which is usually called the M-wave and, if present, a small late F-wave. With repeated stimulation, the M-wave remains constant but the amplitudes and latencies of the F-wave responses vary.

It follows that if the stimulus site is moved proximally, the latency to the M-wave response will increase but that to the F-waves will be shorter since the total distance travelled by them will be shorter.

Diagram 17.1 illustrates this.

A normal example is shown in Figure 17.1.

In the left-hand pane are the traces from 16 consecutive stimulations which are shown superimposed in the right-hand pane. Please note that the gain in the later sections of each trace is 10 times that of the earlier sections. The values are shown on either side of the dotted vertical line. The sweep speed is given at the top right-hand corner. The stimulus strength is shown above each trace in the left-hand pane. The M-wave response is large and constant whereas the F-waves are small and inconstant.

The variable latency of the F-waves and the difficulty in assessing the conduction distance involved make this a technique which tends to provide more aesthetic than diagnostic satisfaction. However, it may be of some help when investigating a patient with a widespread but predominantly proximal demyelinating neuropathy.

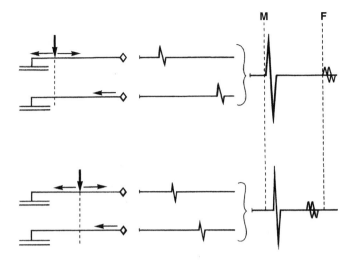

Diagram 17.1 The latency to the small, inconstant F-waves shortens as the stimulus site is moved proximally. (Image included with permission from the Sheffield Teaching Hospitals NHS Foundation Trust.)

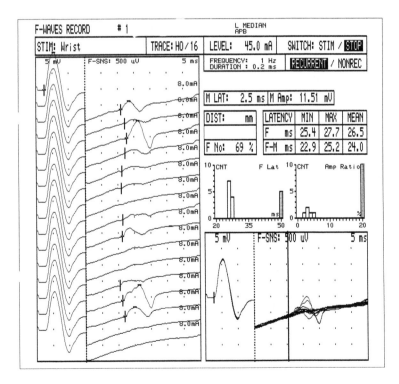

Figure 17.1 A normal F-wave study. (Image included with permission from the Sheffield Teaching Hospitals NHS Foundation Trust.)

H-reflex Studies

As we have seen in Chapter 3, 'Peripheral Nerves; Sensory Nerves', the largest diameter fibres within the peripheral nervous system are the 1a afferents from muscle spindles. In theory, and sometimes in practice, this should make them the first to be depolarised by a weak stimulus. If successfully stimulated in isolation, the wave of depolarisation will travel antidromically and orthodromically. Antidromically, it effectively reaches a dead end since these are sensory fibres to spindles not motor fibres. Orthodromically, the depolarisation is relayed monosynaptically to the anterior horn cell pool supplying the muscle causing it to contract – the electrical equivalent of the tendon reflex. The result is a late, small CMAP known as the H-reflex. This is shown in Diagram 17.2.

As the stimulus strength is slowly increased, from **A** to **B**, we see a gradual increase in the size of the H-reflex as more spindle afferents are stimulated and more anterior horn cells are activated. When the stimulus becomes sufficient to depolarise the motor nerves as well as the Ia afferents, as in **C**, a small CMAP of normal latency appears, the M-wave. Thereafter a very little increase in stimulus strength, shown in **D**, increases the size of the M-wave and continues the obliteration of the H-reflex the beginnings of which were first seen in **C**. The reason for this is to be found in the sequence of nerve depolarisation and repolarisation. As described in Chapter 4, 'Peripheral Nerve Function', after a nerve has been depolarised, it enters a short phase of absolute refractoriness. The orthodromically conducted potential which has produced the M-wave also travels antidromically and meets the orthodromic motor nerve potentials generated by the anterior horn cell for the H-reflex. As each set of action potentials collides, they enter the other's absolute refractory period and cancel out.

Triceps surae is commonly used for this study, as shown in Figure 17.2. Ensuring that the active electrode is over the end-plate zone in such a lengthy muscle can be difficult. In this

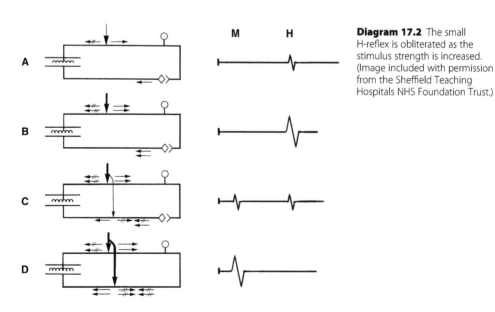

M   **H**

Diagram 17.2 The small H-reflex is obliterated as the stimulus strength is increased. (Image included with permission from the Sheffield Teaching Hospitals NHS Foundation Trust.)

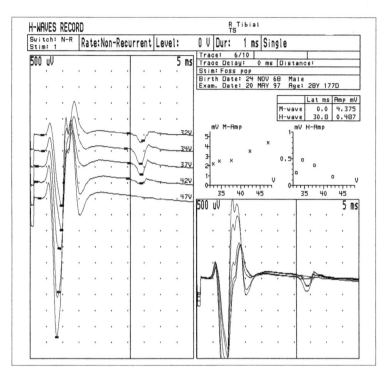

Figure 17.2 A normal H-reflex study. (Image included with permission from the Sheffield Teaching Hospitals NHS Foundation Trust.)

case, it is the indifferent electrode which is close to but not directly over the end-plate zone. As a result, the major component of the CMAP is downward (i.e. positive), and is preceded by a small upward, negative wave. (A mirror image of this response, obtained by reversing the electrode positions, would similarly indicate that the active electrode was not directly over the end-plate zone because there would be a small positive wave preceding the principal negative response. See 'Chapter 7, 'Some Technical Matters; Amplifiers'.)

The gain is shown in the top left-hand corner of both panes and the sweep speed in the top right-hand corner. The results from successive stimuli of increasing strength, as indicated by the voltage value above the terminal portion of each trace, are displayed in the left pane. Initially, a small H-reflex is seen, which increases in amplitude at first before being obliterated as the stimulus strength is increased. On the right side, above the superimposed traces are two small graphs. The left one shows how the amplitude of the M-wave gradually increases with stimulus strength, whereas the right one charts the corresponding rise, fall and ultimate abolition of the H-reflex.

Unfortunately, it is usually the case that despite careful attention to technical factors, particularly stimulus strength and duration (it is claimed that a constant voltage stimulus of long duration is the most effective approach), the test is seldom useful. Certainly, this is the author's experience but others have reported prolonged H-wave latency in S1 root lesions, for example.

18

Clinical Applications

We now look at how these principles are applied in clinical practice.

Myopathy

As described earlier in Chapter 10, 'Electromyography (EMG); Myopathy and Neuropathy', the finding of abnormally short-duration motor unit potentials points to the presence of muscle disease. A very rare, alternative cause of these findings is that of a twig neuropathy which will be discussed in Chapter 19, ' Other Stuff: Aberrant Nerve Pathways, A-waves, EMG Anomalies'. Fibrillation potentials are occasionally seen in cases of polymyositis or inclusion body myositis but unless myotonia is present, implying a disorder such as myotonic dystrophy or myotonia congenita, further refinement of the diagnosis will require a detailed family history probably supplemented by muscle biopsy, and possibly by metabolic and genetic testing. Because myopathy is a patchy disorder, false negative results are common. Disorders affecting type 2 fibres, such as steroid induced myopathy, are invariably associated with normal findings because, as described in Chapter 9, 'Pathology; Muscle', the motor units which are recruited first during voluntary effort are populated with type 1 muscle fibres.

Neuromuscular Transmission Defects

The techniques described in Chapter 16, 'Tests of Neuromuscular Transmission', differentiate between pre-synaptic and post-synaptic disorders. Additional diagnostic testing may involve screening for a thymoma in myasthenia gravis and for small cell cancer in Lambert–Eaton myasthenic syndrome.

Neuropathy

In diagnosing neuropathy, we rely on the principles described in Chapter 10, 'Electromyography (EMG)', Chapter 13, 'Nerve Conduction Studies: Degeneration' and Chapter 14, 'Nerve Conduction Studies: Demyelination', namely, that demyelinating lesions cause slowed and/or desynchronised nerve conduction or conduction block, and degenerating lesions cause reduced SNAPs and/or EMG changes of denervation and regeneration.

First, we will look at generalised peripheral neuropathy, then lesions of some solitary peripheral nerves, and finally proximal lesions.

Generalised Peripheral Neuropathy

We start by considering the effects of widespread pathology within the peripheral nervous system known as peripheral neuropathy or generalised peripheral neuropathy. Depending on whether the principal focus is on the axon or the myelin, we have two major categories, namely, degenerating or demyelinating peripheral neuropathy, respectively.

Peripheral Neuropathy: Degenerating

In a generalised degenerating peripheral neuropathy, sensory nerve pathology is shown by a reduction in the amplitude of the SNAPs, and motor nerve pathology by changes on electromyography. The abnormalities begin distally spreading proximally with disease progression, the so-called dying back process.

As we have seen in Chapter 13, 'Nerve Conduction Studies: Degeneration', maximal conduction velocity is affected modestly if at all. The degree of reduction in SNAP amplitudes is a measure of the degree of pathology. Similarly, as described in Chapter 10, 'Electromyography (EMG)', changes on electromyography include spontaneous activity such as fibrillation and positive sharp waves. There is usually evidence of motor nerve regeneration in the form of MUPs which are increased in duration and possibly polyphasic in form. The degree of motor nerve degeneration can be inferred from the amount by which the recruitment pattern is reduced.

In Figure 18.1 we see recruitment patterns and a sensory study from a patient with a generalised degenerating peripheral neuropathy.

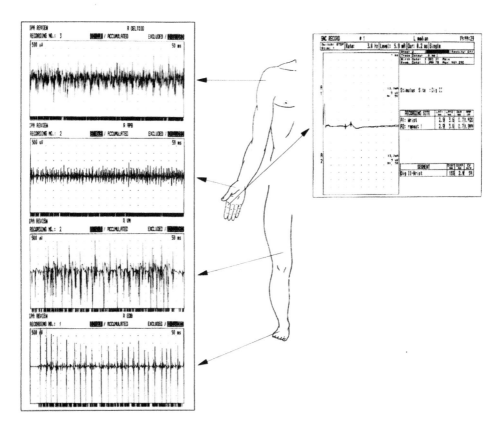

Figure 18.1 Generalised degenerating peripheral neuropathy showing distally predominant motor and sensory nerve abnormalities. (Image included with permission from the Sheffield Teaching Hospitals NHS Foundation Trust.)

The recruitment pattern is normal in deltoid but in all other muscles the patterns are reduced particularly in the leg and especially distally. The median SNAP amplitude is reduced but the maximal sensory conduction velocity is normal. A SNAP could not be recorded from the sural nerve.

These changes represent a generalised degenerating peripheral neuropathy of moderate to marked degree.

Peripheral Neuropathy: Demyelinating

This type of neuropathy is characterised by patchy, slowed conduction in sensory and/or motor fibres. As we have seen in Chapter 14, 'Nerve Conduction Studies: Demyelination', depending on the degree of change and the type and diameter of affected fibres, any or all of the following may occur: increased distal latencies, reduced maximal conduction velocities, desynchronised potentials, conduction block and delayed F-wave latencies.

The degree and extent of the slowing is a measure of the degree of pathology but, as noted in Chapter 9, 'Pathology', severe demyelination will lead to axonal degeneration and therefore its associated electrophysiological abnormalities.

Figure 18.2 of a median nerve motor study shows slowed maximal motor conduction velocity and evidence of conduction block, particularly over the axilla-to-elbow segment.

In Figure 18.3 there is another median motor study, this time showing slight slowing of maximal motor conduction velocity between elbow and wrist but marked desynchronisation of the CMAP over the same segment implying that the brunt of the pathology is falling upon smaller diameter fibres within this section of the nerve. There is probably little if any demyelination between axilla and elbow because the conduction velocity over this segment is within normal limits and the form of the CMAP does not change when the stimulus site is moved from the elbow to the axilla.

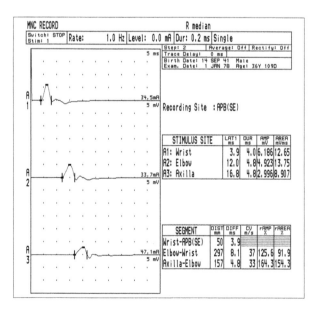

Figure 18.2 Generalised demyelinating peripheral neuropathy showing slowing and conduction block in the median motor study. (Image included with permission from the Sheffield Teaching Hospitals NHS Foundation Trust.)

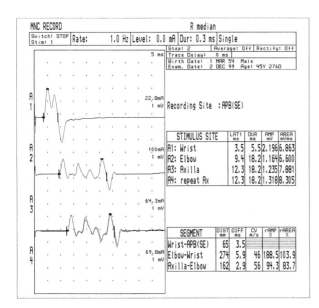

Figure 18.3 Generalised demyelinating peripheral neuropathy showing slowing in all fibres especially the smaller diameter ones in the median motor study. (Image included with permission from the Sheffield Teaching Hospitals NHS Foundation Trust.)

A delayed F-wave latency may occasionally be useful in revealing slowed conduction over the proximal segment of a nerve. Figure 18.4 shows an example of a normal peroneal nerve F-wave study.

And in Figure 18.5 we see a delayed F-wave. Note that the sweep speed is slower to ensure no even later components are missed:

Solitary Peripheral Nerve Lesions

We now consider the diagnostic approach to a selection of frequently encountered peripheral nerve lesions.

Median and Ulnar Entrapment Neuropathies

Features of carpal tunnel syndrome and ulnar nerve entrapment at the elbow have been described in some detail as illustrative examples in Chapter 14, 'Nerve Conduction Studies: Demyelination'.

Chronic compression produces demyelination and although there is evidence that all nerve fibre diameters are susceptible, the largest ones seem to be the most affected. This is fortunate since it is these which tend to be the focus of our examinations.

Sensory testing is usually more sensitive than motor testing in carpal tunnel syndrome, particularly if measurements can be confined to the palm-to-wrist segment as described in Chapter 14, 'Nerve Conduction Studies: Demyelination; Localisation of the Lesion'. Motor studies rely on the demonstration of a prolonged distal latency to abductor pollicis brevis. A problem here is that there is a wide variation in normal measurements, probably due to variations in the underlying anatomy such as the length of the unmyelinated nerve terminals. Having said that, very occasionally an increased distal latency is the only abnormality found in carpal tunnel syndrome. This has been attributed to a separate, and in this case susceptible, compartment within the carpal tunnel for the motor branch of the median nerve.

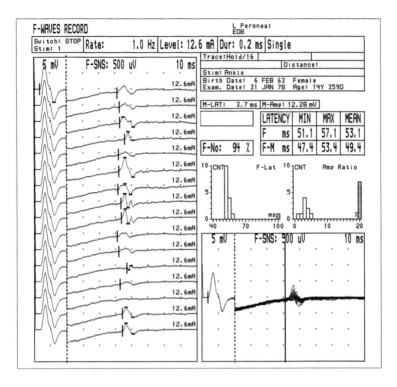

Figure 18.4 A normal F-wave study to extensor digitorum brevis. (Image included with permission from the Sheffield Teaching Hospitals NHS Foundation Trust.)

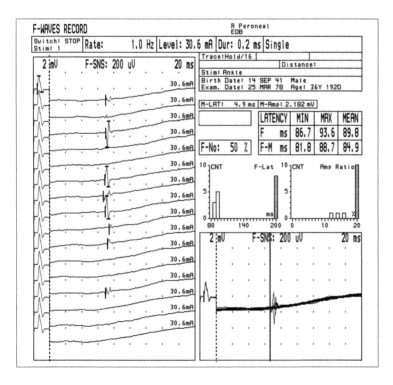

Figure 18.5 A prolonged F-wave latency to extensor digitorum brevis in a generalised demyelinating peripheral neuropathy. (Image included with permission from the Sheffield Teaching Hospitals NHS Foundation Trust.)

In the case of ulnar entrapment at the elbow, measurement of sensory conduction across the lesion can be technically difficult and so motor studies are generally more informative.

This may be the appropriate point to insert a caveat about the prognosis in carpal tunnel syndrome. Patients are often told that decompression will restore normality quickly if not instantaneously. It is true that a mildly compressed nerve in which the pathophysiology is a combination of ischaemia and at most modest demyelination will conduct normally soon after compression is released. If there is more substantial demyelination, recovery by the relatively fast process of remyelination should be measured in days or weeks. But if the lesion has progressed to degeneration, recovery will be slow. A time course of many months is not unusual and an incomplete recovery not uncommon.

Peroneal Nerve Lesions

The peroneal nerve is also susceptible to problems in relation to a joint, this time the knee. As the nerve wraps around the head of the fibula, it divides into the deep peroneal branch supplying tibialis anterior, and the superficial peroneal branch supplying peroneus longus and also incorporating sensory fibres. Compression, causing local demyelination, does occur and needle electrode studies may show some local slowing in sensory and/or motor fibres. However, the author's impression is that degeneration is the predominant pathology rather than demyelination, suggesting that percussion or stretch may be the principal causative factor.

Measurement of motor conduction velocity across the head of the fibula, the site of most lesions of this nerve, can be technically difficult using surface stimulating electrodes to deliver a supramaximal stimulus to the nerve in the popliteal fossa.

Figure 18.6 shows a relatively rare example of slowed motor conduction across the head of the fibula, here between fossa poplitea and capitulum fibulae. There is also evidence of conduction block.

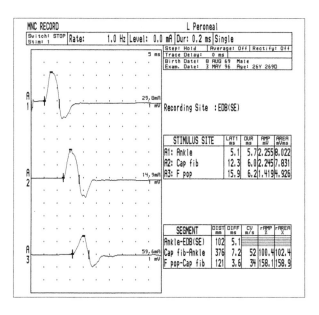

Figure 18.6 Peroneal motor nerve study showing slowed conduction and some conduction block across the head of the fibula. (Image included with permission from the Sheffield Teaching Hospitals NHS Foundation Trust.)

However, in the majority of cases, motor conduction is normal. The diagnosis rests on demonstrating an absent SNAP at the head of the fibula on the affected side in the context of a normal response in the other leg and also a normal sural SNAP on the affected side. This provides evidence of a peroneal nerve lesion as opposed to a lesion within the sciatic nerve or lumbosacral plexus. Further localisation and assessment of the degree of pathology is determined by electromyography.

In Figure 18.7, there is a normal peroneal SNAP on the unaffected side but an absent or at the very best a markedly reduced and indistinct potential on the affected side. In this limb, a reduced recruitment pattern in peroneus longus is also present, together with motor unit potentials of increased duration in tibialis anterior. Conditions outside the peroneal nerve territory were normal.

Radial Nerve Lesions

The majority of lesions of this nerve are due to trauma which is either acute, for example after fracture of the humerus, or subacute, for example as in 'Saturday night palsy'. In other words, there may be some local demyelination but mostly the pathology comprises axonal degeneration.

So, as with peroneal nerve lesions, slowing of motor conduction velocity may sometimes be demonstrated, for example, across the spiral grove, but more often these studies are normal. The diagnosis usually rests on the demonstration of a reduced or absent radial SNAP (by stimulating the superficial branch of the nerve distally and recording antidromically over the first dorsal interspace) and then localising the level of the lesion by sampling progressively more proximal muscles, namely, extensor digitorum communis, brachioradialis and triceps brachii. A posterior interosseous nerve lesion will show abnormalities confined to the extensor muscles of the forearm such as extensor digitorum communis.

Tarsal Tunnel Syndrome

Fortunately from our point of view (and reputation), compression of the distal branches of the posterior tibial nerve in the tarsal tunnel is a fairly rare condition, though it probably exists more often than it is diagnosed electrophysiologically. One would expect that chronic compression of the medial and/or lateral plantar nerves in the tarsal tunnel would show evidence of locally slowed conduction. Whilst this may occur, it is usually the case that the diagnosis rests on the demonstration of axonal degeneration by means of electromyography.

Unfortunately, sensory testing is virtually impracticable. Motor studies are relatively easy but seldom ring the bell.

Shown in Figure 18.8 is a normal latency from medial malleolus to abductor hallucis.

In contrast, in Figure 18.9 we see a prolonged latency and also a markedly desynchronised CMAP showing extremely late components. The amplitude is also reduced. (Note the slower sweep speed and increased gain.) This is an uncommon but eagerly sought experience since the best one can do otherwise is demonstrate evidence of denervation in an affected muscle such as abductor hallucis in the appropriate clinical context and absence of abnormality elsewhere.

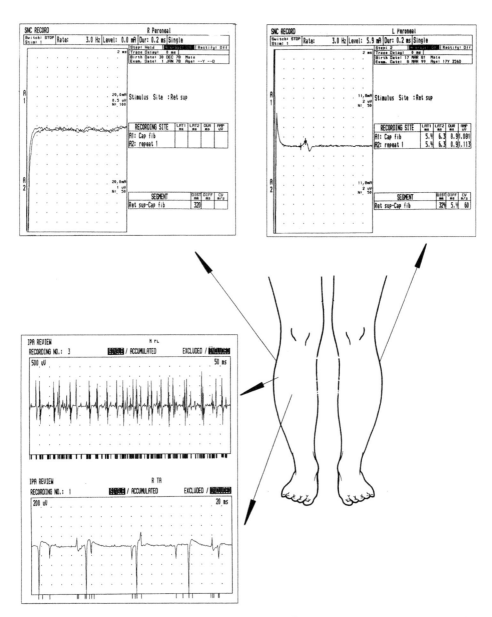

Figure 18.7 Right peroneal nerve lesion. The typical EMG and NCS findings. (Image included with permission from the Sheffield Teaching Hospitals NHS Foundation Trust.)

Figure 18.10 shows an example of tarsal tunnel syndrome where motor unit potentials of increased duration were found in abductor hallucis but conditions in extensor digitorum brevis and elsewhere were normal.

Electromyographers who have visited here know that it is a sensitive area presenting a challenge for the examiner and even more so for the patient.

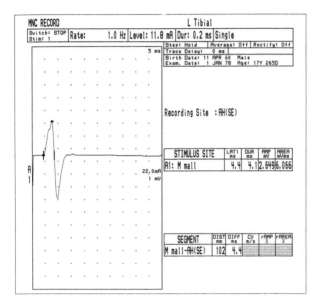

Figure 18.8 Normal latency from medial malleolus to abductor hallucis. (Image included with permission from the Sheffield Teaching Hospitals NHS Foundation Trust.)

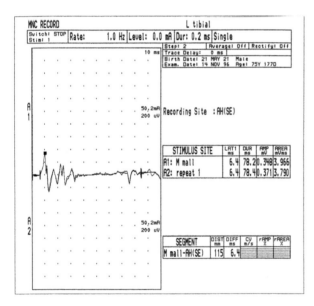

Figure 18.9 Left tarsal tunnel syndrome showing a prolonged distal latency from medial malleolus to abductor hallucis and a markedly desynchronised compound muscle action potential. (Image included with permission from the Sheffield Teaching Hospitals NHS Foundation Trust.)

Proximal Lesions

Radiculopathy

The pathology of these lesions is not well studied. They clearly produce axonal degeneration, which forms the basis of electrophysiological diagnosis. By implication, demyelination may

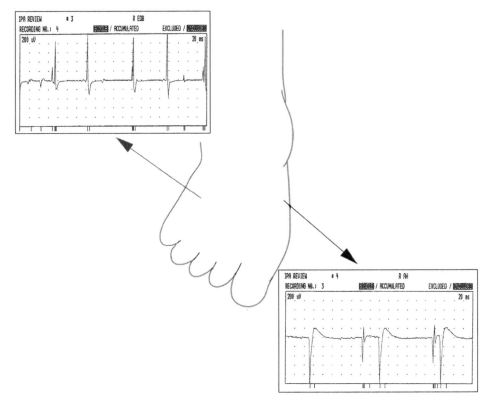

Figure 18.10 Possible right tarsal tunnel syndrome. Motor unit potentials of increased duration in abductor hallucis was the solitary abnormal finding. (Image included with permission from the Sheffield Teaching Hospitals NHS Foundation Trust.)

also occur as evidenced by the finding of slowed H-reflexes in some patients with S1 root lesions.

As we have seen in Chapter 13, 'Nerve Conduction Studies: Degeneration', compression lesions affecting cervical or lumbar nerve roots do not cause changes in the amplitude of SNAPs. The diagnosis of these conditions therefore rests on the demonstration of normal SNAPs and abnormal EMG findings. The distribution of the latter will provide a guide to the level at which nerve root compression is occurring but as limb muscles are always innervated by nerves containing contributions from at least two roots, localisation by these means is poor. In theory, this obstacle can be overcome by examining paraspinal muscles which often receive their nerve supply from a single root, but even here abnormalities may extend beyond a single myotome. In these muscles, fibrillation potentials and positive sharp waves are sought. Difficulties can arise in distinguishing them from so-called atypical end-plate potentials.

In Figure 18.11, we see normal MUPs in right deltoid and right abductor pollicis brevis but MUPs of increased duration, indicating motor nerve regeneration and thus prior degeneration, in right extensor digitorum communis and in right flexor digitorum

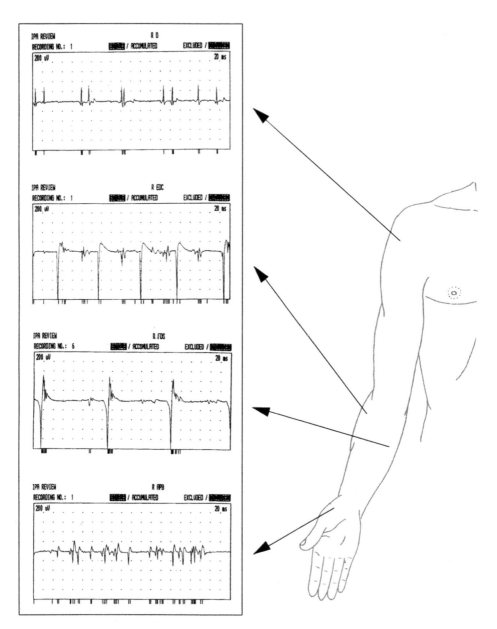

Figure 18.11 Cervical radiculopathy. Motor units of increased duration in right extensor digitorum communis and right flexor digitorum superficialis associated with normal sensory studies. (Image included with permission from the Sheffield Teaching Hospitals NHS Foundation Trust.)

superficialis. In the context of normal sensory studies, these changes imply a cervical radiculopathy affecting the C7 and/or C8 nerve roots.

It should be understood that the value of these studies is to indicate the presence of a radiculopathy rather than to localise it.

Thoracic Outlet Syndrome

In theory, the syndrome causes chronic compression and thus local demyelination. F-wave testing should come into its own here but seldom does. The reason is simple: if the lesion is demyelinating we are probably looking for a delay of no more than a few milliseconds. The normal variation in F-wave latencies is considerable. As we have seen in Chapter 17, 'Other Techniques: F-waves and H-reflexes', in a given individual, this is due in part to the prevailing state of anterior horn cell excitability and also to the normal range of nerve conduction velocities. Even when attempts to allow for these factors are taken into account, abnormalities may be elusive.

The diagnosis is therefore often made at a relatively late stage when many fibres have undergone degeneration. The constellation of findings which will often baffle the novice comprise evidence of denervation in abductor pollicis brevis but frequently not in ulnar-supplied intrinsic muscles of the hand coupled with a normal median nerve SNAP but a reduced or absent ulnar nerve SNAP. However, much earlier diagnosis may be supported by the finding of a reduced SNAP recorded from the medial antebrachial cutaneous nerve which is composed of fibres from the T1 root.

By the time severe wasting of abductor pollicis brevis has occurred, the diagnosis should be easily reached by a competent clinician without the need for investigation. The initial sparing of ulnar-supplied muscles is said to be due to the fact that the median motor nerve fibres to the hand lie closer to the cervical rib or band.

Chapter 19

Other Stuff: Aberrant Nerve Pathways, A-waves, EMG Anomalies

Revelation of Aberrant Nerve Pathways

The normal human body can exhibit a number of curious structural anomalies and the nervous system is not exempt.

Martin–Gruber Anastomosis

In some normal individuals there is a motor branch of the median nerve which runs to the ulnar nerve in the forearm. It is said to have an incidence of 10–20%.

Martin–Gruber anastomosis is most often detected in the investigation of carpal tunnel syndrome. Typically, there is a prolonged distal latency but the maximal motor conduction velocity between elbow and wrist is abnormally fast. This is because the conduction time from elbow to muscle within the anastomotic fibres is not delayed at the wrist. The other give away is that a CMAP recorded with surface electrodes will show an initial positive deflection when the nerve is being stimulated at the elbow, indicating that the potential is being generated some distance from the end-plate region of abductor pollicis brevis.

An example is shown in Figure 19.1.

Accessory Deep Peroneal Nerve

Usually, extensor digitorum brevis is supplied by the terminal portion of the deep peroneal nerve, but it can receive some of its nerve supply from the accessory deep peroneal nerve which arises from the superficial peroneal nerve and then passes behind the lateral malleolus before supplying the muscle.

The key to unveiling this variation is the finding of a much larger CMAP when stimulating at capitulum fibulae compared with the amplitude of the CMAP when stimulating the distal part of the deep peroneal nerve at the ankle. If the stimulating electrodes are placed just behind the lateral malleolus, a nice, big CMAP will be seen. The combined amplitudes of these CMAPs obtained during distal stimulation should approximate the amplitude of the CMAP elicited during proximal stimulation. An example is shown in Figure 19.2.

Axon Reflex or A-wave

Occasionally, when performing F-wave studies a so-called A-wave appears between the early, direct M-response and the F-waves. This has also been called an axon reflex although it is nothing to do with the vascular reflex of the same name. It is thought to be due to a regenerating motor nerve branch. When a distally applied stimulus moves antidromically

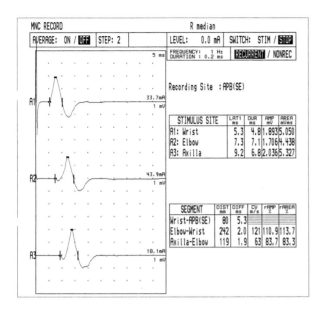

Figure 19.1 Martin–Gruber anastomosis in a patient with carpal tunnel syndrome. (Image included with permission from the Sheffield Teaching Hospitals NHS Foundation Trust.)

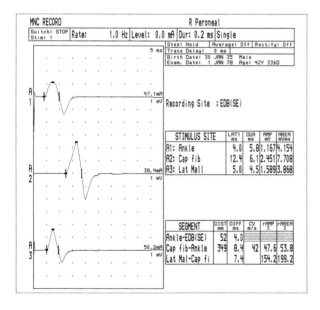

Figure 19.2 An accessory peroneal nerve. (Image included with permission from the Sheffield Teaching Hospitals NHS Foundation Trust.)

along motor nerves, it passes the junction from which this nerve branch originates. The regenerated nerve becomes depolarised and conducts orthodromically back to the muscle. The response is therefore stable and consistent, contrasting with the intermittent F-waves of variable latency reflecting the varying excitability of the anterior horn cells. An alternative

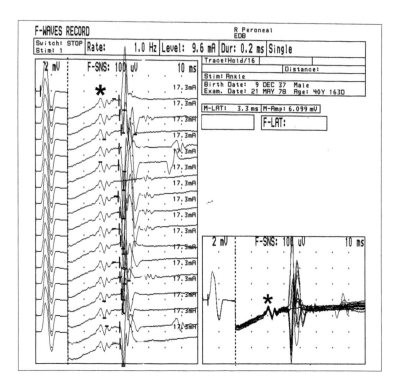

Figure 19.3 An axon reflex. The A-wave (denoted by an asterisk) is constant in latency, amplitude and form distinguishing it from the later F-wave. (Image included with permission from the Sheffield Teaching Hospitals NHS Foundation Trust.)

explanation of the A-wave is that demyelination causes ephaptic or side-to-side depolarisation between nerve fibres.

In the study shown in Figure 19.3, there are intermittent and variable F-waves at about 50 ms. There is also a smaller, constant A-wave arising at just less than 40 ms, denoted by the asterisk.

EMG Anomalies

Neuropathy Masquerading as Myopathy

The left-hand section of Diagram 19.1 shows three normally innervated muscle fibres.

The end-plate zone is depicted by the dotted lines. As described in Chapter 10, 'Electromyography (EMG); Myopathy and Neuropathy', the duration of the MUP will depend on the temporal dispersion of the individual muscle action potentials at the recording electrode and, therefore, the spatial dispersion of the end-plates; that is, the width of the end-plate zone.

The right-hand section of the diagram shows the loss of one of these terminal nerve fibres. This leads to a narrower end-plate zone and hence an MUP of shorter duration. In other words, a neuropathy has produced the EMG appearance of a myopathy. This rare finding is caused by a so-called twig neuropathy which is said to occur, for example, in alcoholic neuropathy.

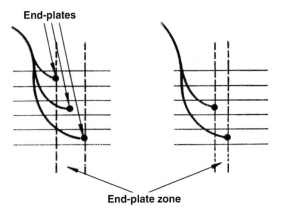

End-plates

End-plate zone

Diagram 19.1 A twig from a peripheral nerve ending has degenerated resulting in a smaller end-plate zone, leading to a motor unit potential of reduced duration. (Image included with permission from the Sheffield Teaching Hospitals NHS Foundation Trust.)

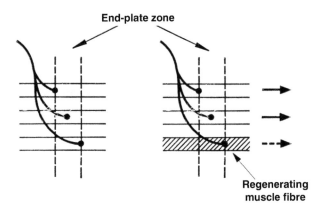

End-plate zone

Regenerating muscle fibre

Diagram 19.2 Conduction in regenerating muscle fibres is abnormally slow leading to a motor unit potential of increased duration. (Image included with permission from the Sheffield Teaching Hospitals NHS Foundation Trust.)

Myopathy Masquerading as Neuropathy

Once again, we imagine three normally innervated muscle fibres as shown in the left-hand section of Diagram 19.2.

In the right-hand section, the hatching represents a regenerating muscle fibre. Conduction in such fibres is slowed and so, although there is no change in width of the end-plate zone, the temporal dispersion of the muscle action potentials arriving at the recording electrode will be increased. This leads to an MUP of increased duration mimicking the finding in a neuropathy.

As has been noted earlier, the role of electrophysiology in the diagnosis of myopathy is limited. Having established the presence of this pathology, refinement of the diagnosis will usually depend on other disciplines. More especially, electrophysiological examination is seldom if ever requested to monitor progress, which the author hopes is the explanation for having never consciously seen this phenomenon.

Normal Values

Chapter 20

The terms normal and abnormal have been liberally applied. The limitations of these concepts need to be addressed.

To construct a normal database, a sufficiently large and representative population must be enrolled. Given the invasive technique of electromyography and the anxiety induced by the notion of electrical stimulation in some subjects, this is no easy task. Ethical considerations are especially important. The obstacle presented to paediatric diagnosticians is particularly daunting. Pooling of data is theoretically attractive providing there is strict standardisation of methods. Difficulties in complying with this basic necessity may be the reason why nirvana remains distant.

If an individual clinic is unable to subscribe to a consensus of this kind, it must maintain a consistent technical approach to recording and stimulation, including skin temperature, electrode type and placement, as well as to amplifier settings.

Subject variables, particularly age, are also critical. With advancing years, evidence of subclinical nerve degeneration occurs as reflected in smaller SNAPs and a tendency to slight slowing of maximal conduction velocities. Skin thickness and hydration are also important but difficult to quantitate. Sensory potentials recorded over dry, thick skin will be reduced in amplitude in proportion to the degree of the greater impedance these factors introduce. If the subject is obese, the increased distance between a nerve and a surface recording electrode could lead to a reduction in the amplitude of the SNAP or MNAP. In extreme cases, the scope of electromyography of proximal muscles may be reduced.

A normal finding can often be inferred from its association with a clear, circumscribed lesion elsewhere. An asymptomatic contralateral limb frequently provides invaluable internal control data. Feedback from referring clinicians also allows retrospective re-evaluation of measurements. Cumulative experience is invaluable. During apprenticeship, the trainee is able to build on the knowledge of the tutor.

On the other hand, we should guard against over-interpretation of results. It may be true that a given value, measured to sixteen decimal places and corrected for normal temperature and pressure, lies just outside (an arbitrary) statistical confidence limit. But is it likely to be clinically relevant? Clinicians unfamiliar with reports on electromyography and nerve conduction studies should be helped to evaluate such data. This is yet another reason for the investigator to have a solid grounding in clinical neurology.

These difficulties will probably be solved differently in different clinics. Nevertheless, the attempt to build a normal database, at least for the most commonly used techniques, should be encouraged. Where such data remain deficient, the diagnostic conclusion should not necessarily be discarded. Most neurologists rely on an assessment of the briskness or otherwise of tendon reflexes. The author has yet to see one consult a normal database before pronouncing the outcome.

Chapter 2

Conclusion

We began by posing some diagnostic questions:
- What is the location of the disorder? (Is it in muscle, nerve or the neuromuscular junction, and if nerve, is the condition local or widespread?)
- What is the pathology? (If muscle is affected, can it be defined? If nerve, is it degenerating or is it demyelinating?)
- What is the severity and thus the prognosis? (What is the degree of change? And what is the likely clinical diagnosis and thus prognosis?)
- Having identified an abnormality, can it be monitored?

Localisation and Pathology

It is convenient to consider these two together.

Myopathy

Electromyography is used to diagnose abnormalities within muscle tissue and will help to distinguish between myopathy and neuropathy. In myopathy there are motor unit potentials of reduced duration and, until a late stage, a full recruitment pattern. However, unless myotonia is present signifying one of the clinical forms of this condition, the diagnosis of the specific pathology will rest on other factors such as clinical presentation, muscle biopsy and genetic factors.

Neuropathy

By contrast, electromyographic changes arising as a result of neuropathy show motor unit potentials of increased duration and a reduced recruitment pattern. Fasciculation points to an anterior horn cell disorder.

The location of neuropathic lesions by means of nerve conduction studies is inextricably linked to the nature of the underlying pathology.

Demyelination causes focal slowing over the affected region as shown by any of the following: reduced maximal motor conduction velocity; reduced maximal sensory conduction velocity; increased distal latency; abnormal desynchronisation of CMAPs, SNAPs or MNAPs. In extreme cases, there will be conduction block.

Degeneration causes no more than modest slowing of conduction velocity, if any. A generalised peripheral neuropathy will show distally predominant reduced or absent SNAPs and/or MNAPs. The localisation of focal degenerative disease, as may occur in isolated peripheral nerve disorders or proximal lesions such as plexus lesions or radiculopathy, depends less on abnormal nerve conduction studies and more on the distribution of EMG changes.

Neuromuscular Transmission Disorders

Repetitive nerve stimulation and single-fibre electromyography may be abnormal in disorders of neuromuscular transmission. In myasthenia gravis, where the pathology is post-synaptic there is a decrementing response during repetitive nerve stimulation.

In Lambert–Eaton myasthenic syndrome, in which the pathology is a pre-synaptic, there is also a slight decrementing response at low rates of stimulation but a greatly pronounced incrementing response at high rates of stimulation.

In both types of pathology, single-fibre electromyography may show increased jitter. In severe cases, this is accompanied by blocking. It is a more sensitive though less specific test than repetitive nerve stimulation in these conditions as similar changes may also occur, for example, in peripheral nerve regeneration.

Severity

Electromyography can be very helpful in detecting mild degrees of myopathy but in moderate to severe cases, clinical features will be more informative in gauging severity.

The degree of demyelinating pathology is reflected in the amount of slowed conduction and, ultimately, conduction block. Severely demyelinated nerves are unstable and will undergo distal degeneration.

Measures aimed at quantifying degeneration are helpful rather than precise. In the case of nerve conduction studies, the SNAPs may be reduced in amplitude. But since the normal distribution of these is positively skewed, some cases will not show a definite abnormality until a relatively late stage. Quantification of recruitment patterns remains elusive. Nevertheless, a severely reduced or even moderately reduced pattern will provide some guide to the degree of denervation present.

The amplitude of the CMAP at low rates of stimulation may be reduced in severe abnormalities of neuromuscular transmission. The amount of jitter and blocking is generally a better guide to the degree of compromise.

Monitoring

For a diagnostic specialty based so heavily on numerical data, it has to be said that electromyography's role in monitoring is disappointing. Generally, clinical features are more informative in most conditions.

In the case of myopathy, electrophysiological diagnosis is qualitative not quantitative.

In nerve conduction studies, prolonged distal latencies, slowed conduction velocities and/or abnormally desynchronised potentials as a consequence of demyelination can easily be monitored. But since these changes are often associated with entrapment neuropathy, improvement after decompression seldom needs this kind of confirmation. If they have been caused by a generalised demyelinating neuropathy then sometimes re-testing can be clinically helpful.

Monitoring in cases of nerve degeneration is more difficult. This is partly because changes in amplitude of SNAPs and MNAPs are heavily dependent on the location of stimulating and recording electrodes, and partly because alterations in the degree of pathology need to be quite substantial before they can be detected. If recording conditions are carefully standardised, measurement of SNAP amplitudes may allow monitoring of degenerative conditions but the very slow process of regeneration makes this a more attractive proposal in principle than in practice. Patients receiving neurotoxic medication can be successfully monitored given careful control of electrode placement.

That regeneration after severe nerve degenerative lesions is occurring may sometimes be picked up on electromyography in the form of nascent motor unit potentials. In less severe cases, regenerating nerves producing immature neuromuscular junctions may be detected through increased jitter.

The monitoring of neuromuscular transmission is a standard procedure in theatre when the patient is receiving muscle relaxant during anaesthesia. But electrophysiological monitoring of myasthenia gravis or Lambert–Eaton myasthenic syndrome is seldom requested.

As promised, the summary Table 21.1 tells you what you have been told!

Table 21.1 Summary table (Table 1.1) completed.

Anatomy	Pathology	Neurophysiology	
		EMG	*NCS*
Muscle	Myopathy	SA ↓ MUPD (↑ Recruitment pattern) Polyphasic MUPs	
Neuromuscular junction	MG	Increased jitter	Decrementing response
	LEMS	Increased jitter	Incrementing response
Peripheral nervous system		**D/M Neuropathy**	
	Compression lesions* GPN***		↓ CV ↑DL ↑ Desynchronisation Conduction block
		D/G Neuropathy	
	Peripheral nerve lesions* Plexus lesions** Radiculopathy** GPN***	SA ↑ MUPD ↓ Recruitment pattern Polyphasic MUPs	↓ SNAP (CMAP) Amp (Possible slight ↓ CV)
	AHC disease***	Also fasciculation	

Key to abbreviations:

* Local changes
** Regional changes
*** Widespread changes

MG Myasthenia gravis
LEMS Lambert–Eaton myasthenic syndrome
GPN Generalised peripheral neuropathy
AHC Anterior horn cell disease

D/M Demyelinating
D/G Degenerating

SA Spontaneous activity
MUPD Motor unit potential duration
MUPs Motor unit potentials

CV Conduction velocity
DL Distal latency
SNAP Sensory nerve action potential
CMAP Compound muscle action potential
(Amp = Amplitude)

Glossary

Absolute refractory period. The period after a nerve has fired during which a stimulus of whatever strength is incapable of causing it fire again.

Action potential. A propagated potential generated by an active nerve fibre or muscle fibre.

Afferent nerve. A nerve carrying impulses centrally from the periphery; a sensory nerve.

Alpha motor neuron. A large anterior horn cell supplying extrafusal muscle fibres.

Annulospiral receptors. Nerve endings wrapped around the central part of the muscle spindle providing information about the length of the muscle.

Anterior horn cell. A nerve cell located in the ventral (anterior) horn of the spinal grey matter supplying a muscle.

Antidromic. Running in the opposite direction to normal, physiological travel.

Axon. The nerve emanating from the nerve cell body, the soma.

Bipolar. see Soma.

Cannula. Here used to refer to the barrel of a hollow needle.

Capacitance. The amount of electric charge stored by a conductor.

Collateral re-innervation. The re-innervation of denervated muscle fibres by nearby normal nerve fibres which develop collateral sprouts.

Compound muscle action potential. The summation of all the muscle action potentials generated by motor nerve stimulation.

Continuous conduction. Nerve conduction in unmyelinated fibres. The nerve action potential travels along the nerve from one sodium channel to the next.

Dendrite. Small projections on a neuron to which terminals from other nerves attach.

Depolarisation. A reduction of the resting membrane potential.

Distal. Further or furthest from the centre (which can be considered to be the spinal column).

Dorsal root. Each spinal nerve has two roots, a ventral one and a dorsal one. The dorsal root contains sensory fibres travelling into the spinal cord.

Dying-back neuropathy. Axonal neuropathy extending centripetally from the extremities.

Efferent nerve. A nerve carrying impulses to the periphery; a motor nerve.

End-plate zone or region. The mid-point of a muscle to which its nerve supply is attached.

Ephaptic transmission. Lateral transmission between adjacent nerve or muscle fibres.

Exocytosis. The active discharge of a molecule from a cell.

Extrafusal muscle fibres. The fibres within a muscle which produce movement and/or tension.

Flower spray endings. Nerve endings attached to the distal parts of the muscle spindle providing information about the length of the muscle.

Golgi tendon organ. Nerve endings attached to a tendon providing information about the tension generated.

Impedance. The opposition of a structure to the flow of a time-varying current.

Initial segment. The most proximal segment of a motor nerve. It contains a high density of sodium channels and is therefore the site at which the nerve action potential is initiated.

Intrafusal muscle fibres. The small fibres within a muscle containing sensory nerve endings which signal the amount and rate of change of muscle length. Also known as muscle spindles.

Ischaemia. An inadequate blood supply.

Latency. The delay between the delivery of a stimulus and the onset of the response. Proximal and distal stimuli generate proximal and distal latencies, respectively.

Membrane potential. An active process by which the interior of a cell is negatively charged relative to the exterior. Also known as the resting potential.

Mixed nerve. A nerve containing sensory and motor fibres.

Monopolar. see Soma.

Monosynaptic. A junction between only two neurons.

Motor unit. The anterior horn cell, its peripheral nerve and all the muscles fibres it innervates.

Motor unit action potential. The combined muscle action potentials belonging to a single motor unit.

Muscle action potential. The propagated action potential generated by an active muscle fibre.

Muscle spindles. See Intrafusal muscle fibres.

Myelin. The component of an insulating sheath around an axon.

Myotome. The group of muscles innervated by a single spinal nerve.

Nerve action potential. The propagated potential generated by an active nerve fibre.

Neuron. A nerve.

Node (of Ranvier). The small gap between adjacent segments of myelin which exposes the axon where abundant voltage-gated sodium channels are present.

Orthodromic. Running in the same direction as normal, physiological travel.

Paraspinal muscles. Muscles located along the vertebral column, adjacent to its spinous process.

Plexus. An area where sensory and motor fibres mingle and recombine to form peripheral nerves.

Polyphasic motor unit potential. A motor unit action potential with five or more phases.

Proximal. Nearer or nearest to the centre (which can be considered to be the spinal column).

Radiculopathy. Pathology within the spinal nerve roots, usually mechanically induced, as they pass through the foramina between adjacent vertebrae.

Relative refractory period. The period after a nerve has fired during which it may fire again but only if the stimulus strength is greater than that of the original stimulus.

Repolarisation. A restoration of the resting membrane potential following depolarisation.

Resting potential. See Membrane potential.

Saltatory conduction. Nerve conduction in myelinated fibres. The nerve action potential travels down the nerve by jumping from one node of Ranvier to the next.

Schwann cells. Cells that lie alongside the axon. They wrap around it to form concentric layers of myelin.

Signal to noise ratio. The ratio of the power of the signal of interest to that of the background noise.

Soma. The nerve cell body from which its nerve arises. The cell is monopolar if the nerve is single and bipolar if double.

Spatial dispersion. Scatter.

Spatial summation. The combined effect of inputs arriving at different locations.

Stimulus artefact. Distortion of a recorded potential caused by the stimulus as seen in nerve conduction studies.

Spike potentials. A rapid increase and decrease in voltage as seen in action potentials.

Sweep speed. The speed at which the display moves across the screen of an oscilloscope.

Synapse. A junction between two nerve cells.

Synaptic vesicles. Membrane-bound spheres containing acetylcholine.

Temporal dispersion. The asynchronous arrival of action potentials which will attenuate the maximal amplitude of their sum depending on its degree.

Temporal summation. The combined effect of inputs arriving at the same location but at different times.

Threshold potential. The potential which must be exceeded for a muscle or nerve fibre to fire thereby generating a propagated action potential.

Triceps surae. The calf muscles comprising the medial and lateral gastrocnemius and the soleus.

Trigger and delay. The display of an oscilloscope is triggered by a potential which can then be revealed in its entirety after a delay from the onset of the sweep.

Ventral root. Each spinal nerve consists of two roots, a ventral one and a dorsal one. The ventral root contains motor fibres travelling from the spinal cord.

Voltage-gated channels. Channels dedicated to the flow of specific ions which open in response to a specified degree of voltage change.

Further Reading

Books on Electromyography and Nerve Conduction Studies

Kimura, Jun. (2013). *Electrodiagnosis in Diseases of Nerve and Muscle: Principles and Practice*. Oxford University Press. (Also deals with evoked potentials)

Michell, Andrew. (2013). *Understanding EMG*. Oxford University Press.

Ferrante, Mark A. (2018). *Comprehensive Electromyography: With Clinical Correlations and Case Studies*. Cambridge University Press.

Preston, David C. and Barbara E. Shapiro (2020). *Electromyography and Neuromuscular Disorders*, 4th ed. Elsevier. (Also deals with ultrasound)

Practical Guides

Leis, A. Arturo and Michael P. Schenk (2013). *Atlas of Nerve Conduction Studies and Electromyography*, 2nd ed. Oxford University Press.

Weiss, Lynn D., Jay M. Wiess and Julie K. Silver (2022). *Easy EMG: A Guide to Performing Nerve Conduction Studies and Electromyography*. Elsevier.

Multi-author Reference Books

Dumitru, Daniel (ed.). (2001). *Electrodiagnostic Medicine*, 2nd ed. Elsevier Health Sciences. (Also deals with evoked potentials, transcranial magnetic stimulation and intraoperative monitoring)

Aminoff, Michael J. (ed.). (2012). *Aminoff's Electrodiagnosis in Clinical Neurology*. Elsevier. (Also deals with evoked potentials and electroencephalography)

Mills, Kerry R. (ed.). (2015). *Oxford Textbook of Clinical Neurophysiology*. Oxford University Press. (Also deals with evoked potentials, electroencephalography, magnetoencephalography and transcranial magnetic stimulation)

Rubin, Devon I. (ed.). (2021). *Clinical Neurophysiology*. Oxford University Press. (Also deals with evoked potentials and electroencephalography)

Index